The Nature of
General Family Practice

The Nature of General Family Practice

583 clinical vignettes in family medicine

An alternative approach to syllabus development

Edited by

W. E. Fabb & J. R. Marshall

Part 4

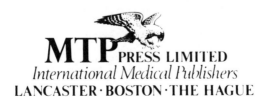

MTP PRESS LIMITED
International Medical Publishers
LANCASTER · BOSTON · THE HAGUE

Published in UK by
MTP Press Limited
Falcon House
Lancaster, England

ISBN 0-85200-726-4

Phototypeset by Blackpool Typesetting Services Ltd.,
Blackpool, Lancashire, England.
Printed by Redwood Burn Ltd.,
Trowbridge

Contents

Preface

The idea of producing this book of case histories from general family practice was only a twinkle in the editors' eyes until October 1980, when in a room in the Marriott Hotel in New Orleans, the editors met with John Fry, Joseph Levenstein and Bill Jackson to discuss new book projects. The idea was put to the group, which endorsed it enthusiastically. Encouraged by this and by John Fry's advice, the conception of *The Nature of General Family Practice* took place.

It was agreed that to illustrate the universal nature of general family practice it would be useful to collect case histories from all around the world, that for preference they should be brief, and that they should be accompanied by major questions and sub-questions, but no answers. The name 'Vignettes' was applied to these cases and their questions.

Subsequently, well over a hundred family physicians were asked by letter to provide ten vignettes. Sixty doctors from ten countries accepted the invitation and forwarded their contributions during the second half of 1981. Almost all of those who, for a variety of reasons were unable to contribute, said they liked the idea and looked forward to using the final product. Altogether, over 600 vignettes were received, and 583 selected for final inclusion.

In order to preserve the flavour of the cases, the editors have made as few changes as were necessary to comply with the format of presentation. The cases represent each contributor's own words, own expressions and own ways of telling a story. They give a feeling for the doctor and the way he or she thinks and feels.

The gestation of this book has been a long one, but the baby looks to be in good shape. Whether it will be an only child, will depend on how people like the look of this one.

W. E. Fabb,
J. R. Marshall,
Melbourne,
1983

CHAPTER 15

Upper Respiratory Problems (Including ENT Problems)

This chapter comprises a series of ear problems, with emphasis on the recognition and management of otitis media; nasal problems, including epistaxis, sinusitis and nasal allergy; mouth and throat problems, including a number of cases of sore throat of varying aetiology; several cases of cough resulting from a variety of causes; and the problem of a bone in the throat. These cases represent some of the most common conditions seen by the family physician.

Ear problems

289 **MATTHEW B.   AGED 2**

Matthew B. had had a cold for the past 24 hours. He had had no previous ear trouble but an hour before being brought to the office, had developed an intense earache affecting his right ear. He was crying and distressed by pain.

1. What clinical examination would you make and how would you do it?
2. What is the most likely diagnosis?
3. What predisposing conditions might be associated with this disorder?
4. What is the most likely causative organism?
5. What medications would you prescribe?
6. What advice would you give the parents?

H. C. Watts, Perth, Australia

290 **M.N.   AGED 3**

The patient presents with a coryza for 4 days, cough for 2 days and pulling at the ears with disturbed sleep in the previous night. He has had two similar previous attacks. On examination, the temperature is 38 °C, throat slightly red, chest clear. Ears: left drum – shiny, slightly full and injected, right drum – red around the handle, dull drum and bulging a little.

1. What are this child's problems?
2. What immediate treatment is indicated?
3. What advice would you offer to the parents about future management?

T. D. Manthorpe, Port Lincoln, Australia

291 **JOHN F.   AGED 6**

John is brought by his mother. He awoke last night with earache. He has had earaches before. He is chirpy and not in pain. Examination shows a red left ear drum. There is no fever.

1. What is the diagnosis?
2. What would you do?

J. Fry, Beckenham, UK

DAVID M.   AGED 3

292

Doctor M. had built a small cottage at a remote beach. It was about 50 miles over a poor road from the nearest doctor. He had had a busy few weeks and decided not to take his medical bag as he wanted to get away from it all and not be disturbed by medical work.

As they approached the cottage David M. began to complain of a pain in the cheek. He was about 3 years old and his father thought he might be cutting a tooth. Presently the pain worsened and David was very miserable and cried a great deal. Dr. M. had a look as best he could in the mouth but that seemed quite normal. The nose was a little congested but otherwise in the absence of medical equipment, nothing could be found. Eventually a visit to the general store produced an aspirin and David was made sufficiently comfortable to go off to sleep.

In the morning, to his horror Dr. M. discovered a small patch of moisture on David's pillow and there was some pus in the aural canal. David felt much better.

1. Why was the cause not recognized?
2. What treatment would you have recommended if the diagnosis had been made in the first instance?
3. Do you regard otitis media as a medical emergency?
4. Would you wish to follow up the child?

J. G. Richards, Auckland

JAMES H.   AGED 7   SCHOOLBOY

293

James H. developed fever, running nose and cough 4 days ago. The night before last he was very restless and complained of earache and the next morning there was discharge from the right ear and he felt better. This morning he has been vomiting, the earache has returned and he is feverish. He looks sick and the ear is still discharging. He has marked tenderness over his right mastoid.

1. What problems have occurred?
2. How would you manage this problem?
3. Discuss the infection process in this case?

E. J. H. North, Melbourne

MASTER J.R.   AGED 3

294

Master J.R. is brought to you by his mother because of a high temperature last night and today crying incessantly, pulling at both ears and with a rattling chest cough. He has been seen many times over the last 2 years with infections of both ears in association with tonsillitis, and has been hospitalised on a number of occasions at the Children's Hospital for 'bronchitis'.

1. Is this just another attack of otitis media and 'bronchitis'?
2. What do you want to know about the social situation?
3. What long term effects are taking place?

W. F. Glastonbury, Adelaide

295 MRS. S.K. AGED 29 SCHOOLTEACHER

Mrs. S.K. is happily married to an ambitious bank accountant, six years her senior. They have two children: Ronnie aged 3 years, and Susan aged 6 months. She is obviously worried. 'I am sure that Ronnie is partially deaf, doctor' she says.

1. How would you clarify this problem?
2. What are the implications on the family, of a child suffering from permanent hearing impairment?
3. What facilities in the community can assist the family to cope with a child suffering from impaired hearing?
4. Could Ronnie's hearing disorder have been diagnosed at an earlier age, or perhaps been prevented?

M. R. Polliack, Tel-Aviv, Israel

296 MR. C.K. AGED 50 ENGINEER

Mr. C.K., aged 50, is a 'resident engineer' who has recently moved to the practice area to supervise a construction project. He is living on his own in a hotel. He consults with a 10-day history of bilateral deafness associated with an acute upper respiratory catarrh.

When he reports a week later, it is obvious that the medical measures which were instituted have effected no improvement – his deafness is worse than ever.

Physical reassessment gives no reason to alter the original diagnosis, but he now confesses to feeling generally unwell; it is agreed to put him on the sick list.

He wishes to take the opportunity to convalesce at his own home where his wife resides on her own; but this is 400 miles away and he would like to make the trip by air.

When he returns a week later, his deafness is even more marked. It is decided to seek specialist advice.

1. What measures do general practitioners take to enable patients, who are new to a practice, to make the best use of the services they have to offer?

2. Deafness is a relatively common presenting symptom in family medicine. In general, what are common causes of bilateral deafness?
3. Putting a patient on the 'sick list' is a common doctor activity. Viewed in sociological terms, what does this activity entail?

J. D. E. Knox, Dundee

MR. G.   AGED 54   COMPANY DIRECTOR   **297**

Mr. G. presents complaining of an upper respiratory infection. He has not been overseas for the past 5 years and is currently about to fly to Malaysia on business in two weeks. He wants to know what he should do about immunizations. He is particularly worried about the possibility of getting malaria.

1. What advice will you give him related to his current infection?
2. What will you advise him about immunizations in general?
3. What is your advice about malaria prophylaxis?

J. R. Marshall, Adelaide

Nose problems

298 **MR. GERALD M.** **AGED 71** **RETIRED SCHOOLTEACHER**

Mr. M. is brought into your office with a bleeding nose. He has tried to stop it for the last hour. He has had several previous episodes of epistaxis, but all have stopped quickly when he held his nose. He is on treatment for moderate hypertension.

He has his nose covered by a very blood-stained towel and spits out blood clots as you examine him.

1. What are the likely contributing factors to his epistaxis?
2. How would you manage this situation?
3. What follow up will be needed?

W. E. Fabb, Melbourne

299 **G.P.** **AGED 2½**

G.P. transferred from another practice when the family moved house. Past history of severe nose bleeds with one packing (GP) and two cauteries (ENT specialist) and said to have been fully investigated. The child presented with a severe nose bleed and was said to bruise easily.

1. Why is the above history unsatisfactory?
2. What would your next move be toward effective management?
3. What are your intuitive feelings about this story?

W. D. Jackson, Launceston, Australia

300 **MR. C. CHAN** **AGED 46** **CHINESE RICE MERCHANT**

Mr. Chan complained to the doctor that he had noticed a lump in his neck a few weeks ago. He attributed this lump to his recent bout of late nights and heavy smoking. In the last 2 weeks he has also been having recurrent nose bleeds. However, his main worry is the fact that he has been coughing up some dark, bloody sputum. He does not know whether the blood is coming from his nose or from his lungs. He also has a persistent smelly, post-nasal discharge.

Physical examination revealed a firm mass, size 3 cm × 2 cm in the midcervical chain; other lymph nodes were normal. Chest X-ray and peripheral blood smear were normal.

1. What further examination and investigation are required to establish a diagnosis?
2. What is the treatment of choice?
3. What is the prognosis?

N. C. L. Yuen, Hong Kong

MR. N.M.   AGED 41   SAW MILLER

301

This man has a 10-year history of non seasonal recurring 'colds', blocked nose, operation on sinuses and nose by an ENT specialist 3 years ago, an antral wash out 1 year ago and a lack of response to nose drops, antihistamines, and Rynacrom (sodium cromoglycate). The ENT specialist feels no more can be done, but this patient is still dissatisfied and often in considerable discomfort with a blocked, snuffly nose.

1. Is another referral advisable and if so, to whom?
2. Do simple radical antrostomies have a high success rate in chronic sinusitis?
3. Are there any simple measures that may be helpful?

T. D. Manthorpe, Port Lincoln, Australia

MR. F.M.   AGED 42   INSURANCE AGENT

302

Mr F.M. was seen in the office by appointment complaining of nasal stuffiness for several weeks. Following a cold, several weeks previously, there has been continued nasal congestion and a feeling of fullness in the face. There is no significant nasal drainage. A proprietary antihistamine-decongestant helped a little, briefly, a few weeks previous to the appointment.

Past medical history revealed no previous similar symptoms and no allergic history. The only medications have been occasional aspirin for URIs.

Physical examination revealed a 'nasal' speech. On examination of the nose, there was mild redness of all nasal mucous membranes with some mucopurulent drainage from the inferior right nasal passage, mild to moderate tenderness over the right malar region and equivocal transillumination of the right maxillary sinus. Examination of the heart revealed a grade III left precordial systolic murmur and normal rhythm.

1. What would constitute an appropriate differential diagnosis of this man's respiratory symptoms?
2. What are the ramifications of this man's heart murmur?
3. What laboratory procedures would be of most value in assessing this patient's respiratory infection?
4. What are the expected outcomes of a general type screening examination, even for seemingly well-defined, localized problems such as upper respiratory infection?

L. H. Amundson, Sioux Falls, SD, USA

Mouth and throat problems

303 **BETTY R.   AGED 2**

This child presented with a history of fever and anorexia for 2 days. On examination her temperature was 39.9 °C. She had an offensive breath, ulceration of the tongue, mucous membranes and gums, and enlargement of the cervical lymph nodes. She was drooling saliva and was obviously distressed. Her mother said that she absolutely refused to eat and it was very difficult to persuade her to drink anything.

1. What was the most likely cause of her illness?
2. If this condition were due to an infective agent, what other clinical manifestations could be produced by it?

J. G. P. Ryan, Brisbane

304 **MR. Q.R.   AGED 65   RETIRED ENGINEER**

Mr. R. consults his doctor for the second time about an ulcer on his tongue. On looking at the ulcer, the doctor feels quite certain it has undergone malignant change and he is perturbed about the status of a small lump beneath the mandible. Before he can think what to say next, the patient proceeds to tell the doctor how grateful he and his wife are that the doctor had previously pursued the occurrence of his chest pain to the diagnosis of myocardial vascular insufficiency, and how fortunate it was that the doctor persuaded him, almost against their wishes, to agree to by-pass surgery. He never has angina and has been able to do most of the things he wishes in the 20 months since the operation.

1. What is the doctor thinking?
2. What does he say next to the patient?
3. What does he say to the patient's wife, whom he knows will be ringing up after the consultation?

P. L. Gibson, Auckland

305 **DR. P.F.   AGED 32   UNIVERSITY LECTURER**

Dr. P.F. presents with an acutely painful throat which reveals a marked tonsillar exudate. He has recently arrived from overseas to take up a new position. His wife is pregnant and due to be confined in 6 weeks time. They have two other small children. He has a heavy work load and has heard about the debilitating effects of infectious mononucleosis which is endemic in the area.

1. How specific can a general practitioner be when diagnosing viral respiratory infections?
2. What viral infections cause concern during pregnancy?
3. How does a nuclear family cope when the only wage earner in the family is ill?

B. H. Connor, Armidale, Australia

S.P.   AGED 5

306

S.P., a 5 year old male, gives a 2-day history of sore throat and fever. There has been some trouble swallowing, especially solids. The mother reports that the child has been lethargic. An 8 year old sister had a similar problem one week previously, and a 10 year old sister a similar problem two weeks previously. None of the children have had any immunizations.

1. What would be key diagnostic elements in the history and physical examination?
2. What factors would be helpful in making a positive diagnosis?
3. What other physical findings might help confirm or exclude a streptococcal tonsillo-pharyngitis?

L. H. Amundson, Sioux Falls, SD, USA

TRACEY N.   AGED 4

307

Tracey has had up to ten attacks of follicular tonsillitis in the past 8 months. Her appetite is poor, with consequent weight loss. She plays with her friends, but tires easily. The mother says she snores frequently and has marked halitosis. Today she has a severe attack of follicular tonsillitis, temperature 39.6 °C with large cervical glands.

There is a history of a previous convulsion as an infant.

1. How would you manage the present complaint?
2. What advice would you give the parents?
3. Would you refer the patient to an ENT surgeon?

B. M. Fehler, Johannesburg

MASTER A.T.   AGED 8

308

Master A.T. is brought to your office because of a fever and sore throat of 24 hours duration. He is normally quite well. His family are well known to you, and Anthony is rarely sick. Physical examination reveals acute tonsillitis only.

1. What immediate treatment is necessary?
2. When should antibiotics be prescribed in an otherwise healthy child?
3. What signs of complications would you look for?
4. At this age, and with this history, what other diagnoses are likely?
5. Is tonsillectomy indicated? If so, when?

D. U. Shepherd, Melbourne

309 DICK THOMSON   AGED 8   SCHOOLBOY

Dick's mother brings him along saying 'He's got a sore throat again doctor'. Before you can say anything she is demanding antibiotics to fix it quickly and asking about taking his tonsils out. You notice on the card that Dick has had two episodes of sore throat this winter, the second of which was diagnosed as tonsillitis and treated with penicillin.

This time in fact, the main symptoms (and signs) are a runny nose and cough. He is afebrile. His throat is injected with only slight tonsillar enlargement and no pus. There are a few non-tender cervical lymph nodes. Chest, ears and sinuses are clear.

1. Would you prescribe an antibiotic?
2. Would you arrange a tonsillectomy?
3. What other factors are there in managing this case?

R. P. Strasser, Melbourne

310 DAVID P.   AGED 10   SCHOOLBOY

David is brought in by father having had high fever, headache, muscle pains and sore throat for four days.

David was seen two days ago by a partner and was prescribed salicylates and the father was told he had 'flu'.

The father is angry and demands that something more definite is done.

1. What two problems face the doctor?
2. What could be a differential diagnosis of David's condition given the few facts above?

F. Mansfield, Perth, Australia

311 MR. A.J.   AGED 25   UNIVERSITY STUDENT

It is Sunday morning during the local summer holiday. You visit Ahmed J., a 25 year old Middle Eastern postgraduate university student, living with his wife (from the same country) and 2 year old child in their flat. The reason for the visit is Mr. J., who is lying in bed, looking sorry for himself, and complaining of a sore throat. He does not look ill.

You remember a previous visit for a similar situation some 6 months ago, when you felt that Mr. J. was rather introspective. You note a profusion of patent medicines on the dressing table and at his bedside.

The salient positive physical findings are: pulse rate 82/min; temperature 37.8 °C; a diffuse faucial injection, and palpable tender cervical lymph nodes on both sides.

1. What physical diagnoses would you consider to be likely?
2. What problems, real or imaginary, may be inherent in this situation?
3. How would you manage this situation?

J. D. E. Knox, Dundee

MASTER J.R.   AGED 6   SCHOOLBOY   312

J.R. is in his second year of primary school. He presents with a 2 day history of high fever, sore throat and tender enlarged cervical nodes. He had several similar episodes during his pre-school years, but since starting school has been averaging 3–4 attacks per year. He often has an associated earache and on a number of occasions has been noted to have acute otitis media. His mother also reports that he is a mouth breather and often snores while sleeping.

On examination his tonsils are large with pus in the crypts. The anterior triangle cervical nodes are tender and enlarged. The ears and chest are clear. The oral temperature is 39 °C. A throat swab was taken and oral penicillin and an antipyretic prescribed. The child was given a return appointment for three weeks.

1. Is it possible to determine the aetiological agent of an acute upper respiratory infection on the basis of your physical examination?
2. What are the indications for tonsillectomy and adenoidectomy?
3. What is the role of allergy in the hypertrophy of tonsils and adenoids?

R. L. Perkin, Toronto

MASTER Y.L.   AGED 4   ATTENDS NURSERY SCHOOL   313

A four year old boy, Y.L., comes in to see the doctor with a sore throat. This is his third attack within 9 months. He is pyrexial, 37.6 °C, and has enlarged tonsils and palpable tonsillar glands. The tonsils appear to have pus on them. The doctor initiates a 10-day course of penicillin VK.

The mother brings the patient back 4 days later and if anything, the child looks worse but he is not complaining of his throat. The throat looks unchanged on examination. This failure to respond is unlike the previous attacks.

The doctor tells the mother to come back with the child a week later.

He persists with penicillin and analgesics. The mother is distressed and says that 'It's about time the tonsils were taken out'. The doctor explains his conservative approach to tonsillectomy and what he feels may be the diagnosis here. He also says that he will do blood tests then if the child is still 'ill'.

1. What do you understand by the 'problem solving method', 'hypothesis forming', 'hypothesis testing', 'probability diagnosis', 'testing a hypothesis by treatment' and 'time as a diagnostic tool'?
2. What are your indications for tonsillectomy?
3. Why did the doctor prescribe penicillin VK and for the length of time he did?

J. H. Levenstein, Cape Town

314 MRS. J.A.   AGED 26   HOUSEWIFE

Mrs. J.A. was a working class wife in her twenties with four children between the ages of 2 and 8. She had frequently caused problems in the practice by being abusive towards the receptionist and the nurse and by shouting and swearing at her children in the waiting room. She did her best to see each of the three doctors in turn, always referring to the others by their surnames only and attempting to play off one against the other. Each consultation began aggressively and, if it did not result in a prescription, ended equally aggressively. A source of contention was 6 year old Dawn who had frequent upper respiratory tract infections. Each of the partners in turn reassured Mrs. A. about Dawn's symptoms and the fact that they would diminish as she grew older. Mrs. A. was unconvinced. She had had her own tonsils removed in childhood and was of the firm opinion that her daughter would require the same treatment. The doctors stuck to their guns. Mrs. A. frequently travelled with the children to a nearby city to stay with her mother. On one such occasion Dawn developed a sore throat and was taken to the casualty department of a nearby teaching hospital. There she was treated for tonsillitis and arrangements were made for her to be admitted for tonsillectomy. Mrs. A. returned to the practice in triumph with Dawn minus her tonsils.

1. What is the likely nature of Dawn's problems?
2. What are the indications for tonsillectomy?
3. What are the possible reasons for aggression in a patient?
4. What ethical principles govern relationships between medical practitioners?

T. A. I. Bouchier Hayes, Camberley, UK

315 MRS. FLORENCE A.   AGED 71   HOUSEWIFE

Mrs. A. presents rather distressed an hour after having choked on a fish bone. She feels it is stuck in her throat. She persistently tries to cough it out as you examine her. She tells you she has eaten dry bread in an attempt to remove it, without success.

1. How would you assess this patient?
2. How do you examine a patient with a suspected foreign body in the throat?
3. If the symptoms suggest a foreign body in the throat, but none can be detected, what would you do?

W. E. Fabb, Melbourne

Respiratory problems

316 **KUMBURAI M.   AGED ?   TODDLER**

Mrs. M., previously not known, chubby and obviously pregnant, carried Kumburai into the office. She complained he had been coughing for 3 days and wanted an injection to make him better.

On examination the chest was clear, the temperature was 37.4 °C at 10 a.m., and a crusted discharge could be seen about the nostrils. Kumburai weighed 9 kg but Mrs. M. did not know his age. On questioning it turned out that he had been born at the beginning of the rainy season the year before last, which put his age at about 20 months. He looked normally nourished for a year old baby, and his mid arm circumference was 12.5 cm.

Mrs. M. had walked 9 km to bring him to the office.

1. What treatment should Kumburai have?
2. Is Kumburai suffering from anything of extreme danger to him?
3. What should Mrs. M. be told?

R. T. Mossop, Harare, Zimbabwe

317 **JOHN W.   AGED 5   SCHOOLBOY**

This 5 year old boy is brought in by his mother because he has a high fever, is irritable and crying, and is refusing food and fluids.

The child is restless, crying loudly, flushed and sweating.

1. What are the likely causes of his condition?
2. How would you assess this child?
3. What general advice would you give mother?

W. E. Fabb, Melbourne

318 **WILLIAM ANDREWS   AGED 2   INFANT**

William's mother has brought him to see you because from time to time he has bouts of coughing, especially at night. This has been particularly bad over the last 3 days and nights. He has seemed otherwise well and has been sick only once before with croup when he was 8 months old. There is no specific family history although his mother had bronchitis frequently as a child. Physical examination is completely normal.

14

1. What possible diagnoses are you considering?
2. What investigations would you do?
3. How would manage this problem?

R. P. Strasser, Melbourne

MRS. O.R.　　AGED 46　　HOUSEWIFE

319

Mrs. O.R. who has never had a day's illness in her life develops a flu-like illness with a high temperature and a dry, harsh cough.

After 2 days in bed taking aspirin and patent cough medicines a visit is requested as she still feels unwell. Her cough is productive of only scanty sputum but is becoming painful.

She does not look seriously ill but has a temperature of 38 °C, a pulse rate of 90 and some scattered fine crepitations at the right lung base.

1. What is the diagnosis?
2. Is it either desirable or possible to determine the actual infecting agent?
3. Which, if any, antibiotic is indicated?

A. J. Moulds, Basildon, UK

E.P.　　4 YEAR OLD GIRL

320

E.P. has just entered kindergarten. Previously she has lived in the country with her parents. They now live in a suburban area.

E.P. has had a dry cough and fever for five days. The fever comes and goes – at times she is very sick, but may be bright two hours later.

She has been given only an occasional dose of paracetamol in the last week.

1. What diagnostic hypotheses would be in your mind?
2. How would you test your hypotheses?
3. How would you manage the situation?
4. E.P. has a sister, aged eight months. Mother asks if you can prevent her getting the same condition. What would be your reply?

A. Himmelhoch, Sydney

MR. D.E.　　AGED 18　　COLLEGE STUDENT

321

This lad is a member of a visiting football team. There is an epidemic of influenza at this time. He feels a bit cold and has muscle aches. He plays football today. You are called to see him tonight because he has aches and pains in the muscles, cannot get warm and has a dry cough.

You confidently make a diagnosis of influenza and order aspirin 600 mg, four times a day. You are called again 24 hours later – he is much worse.

1. Is your first diagnosis correct?
2. On the second visit, what do you think has happened?

A. Himmelhoch, Sydney

322 DEREK B. AGED 40 CIVIL SERVANT

Derek B. presented with a variety of symptoms, including fever, malaise, and muscular aches and pains which had been present for a few days. Ten days previously he had returned from a holiday in the Mediterranean. On examination he had a temperature of 39 °C, but nothing else of significance.

Derek was well known to the doctor and had consulted him frequently over the years. He held an important position in the civil service but found it difficult to make decisions. There were problems in his marriage for many years and after much hesitation he finally divorced his wife some months ago.

1. What are the main diagnoses that you would consider for this pyrexial episode?
2. What investigations might you order?
3. How does a patient's past history influence the doctor's approach and management?

J. C. Hasler, Oxford

323 MR. D.C. AGED 40 COMPANY EXECUTIVE

Mr. D.C. consults you because of a dry cough for 3–4 weeks. He is embarassed at coming, and only did so to please his wife. He feels well and has lost no weight. He has had no significant past illnesses. He has a wife and two small children, is a rising company executive, and smokes intermittently when he is under stress, up to 30 cigarettes per day. He drinks socially. He feels his wife is ambitious. He suspects he is being groomed for a senior company position, and is trying to improve his performance at work.

1. Should you discuss his obvious embarrassment?
2. What are the likely physical findings in this case?
3. If the physical findings are negative, should a chest X-ray be performed?
4. Should the management include a cough suppressant?

D. U. Shepherd, Melbourne

MR. A.C.   AGED 32   STOREMAN

Mr. A.C. presents because of a persistent dry cough which has been present for over 2 months. He is apparently otherwise well with no previous illnesses of any significance. He works in a warehouse containing machinery and building supplies. He thinks he has lost some weight recently. He smokes 30–40 cigarettes per day, and is trying to give them up.

1. If your physical examination indicates no specific abnormal findings, with the exception of possible weight loss, what are the most likely diagnoses?
2. What investigations are indicated in this case?
3. What would you prescribe for this cough?
4. If the cough proves to be simply related to excessive smoking, how would you handle this problem?

D. U. Shepherd, Melbourne

CHAPTER 16

Breathing Problems

This chapter begins with a series of cases of dyspnoea due to cardiac, respiratory, allergic, haematological and psychological conditions. Then follows a number of cases of asthma of varying origin, respiratory infection and occupational lung disease. Respiratory problems are among the most common conditions seen by the family physician and often provide him with a challenge in diagnosis or management. The latter is especially true with chronic conditions, such as asthma.

Dyspnoea

325 MR. JOHN J.   AGED 75

A 75 year old man presented to his doctor with increasing shortness of breath on exertion and vague pain in the left upper chest for 6 weeks. Otherwise he felt well. The doctor found an area of bronchial breathing in the left upper zone and arranged a chest X-ray.

1. Why should the doctor arrange a chest X-ray?
2. The chest X-ray showed a carcinoma of the bronchus. What would be the doctor's immediate course of action?
3. The chest specialist recommended no treatment. How would the doctor manage the case now?

J. C. Hasler, Oxford

326 THOMAS R.   AGED 62

He is an old friend of the practice. In 1952 you arranged for him to have a partial gastrectomy for a troublesome chronic duodenal ulcer. He is very grateful for the complete relief from pain and dyspepsia.

In the past 3 months he has noted breathlessness on exertion with a tightness in his chest.

He is a relaxed, ungrumbling person but today he complains of general weakness, pins and needles in his feet and a sore mouth.

1. What are the long term complications of partial gastrectomy?
2. Give your assessment of his new symptoms.
3. How would you manage the likely conditions that you discover?

J. Fry, Beckenham, UK

327 MR. & MRS. S.   AGED 64 AND 62   PENSIONERS

Mrs. S. had consulted the GP several times in recent months complaining of body pains, headaches and dizziness. She seemed convinced that there was something seriously wrong with her physically, but investigations all proved negative.

Mr. S. presented several months after his wife had first consulted the GP. He complained of severe effort dyspnoea. Examination, including ECG, was normal except that he looked pale and his Hb was found to be 4 g/dl. He was admitted to hospital where he was found to have G.I. bleeding.

1. What was the best way of managing Mrs. S.?
2. What was the cause of Mr. S's symptoms?
3. Was there any connection between Mrs. S's symptoms and those of her husband?
4. How are Mr. and Mrs. S. likely to present in the future?

S. Levenstein, Cape Town

MR. J.G.   AGED 76   **328**

This elderly gentleman had been treated for hypertensive heart disease and late onset asthma. His dyspnoea increased for no very obvious reason. Blood examination revealed significant anaemia. In searching for a cause of this a filling defect was found in his caecum during a barium enema.

1. Should surgery be performed?
2. Would you discuss the whole problem with the patient?
3. How could he be offered the best hope for successful surgery if that is the chosen option?

W. D. Jackson, Launceston, Australia

MRS. I.S.   AGED 45   **329**

This mother of 3 teenagers, who works with the local Crisis Centre and currently has a contractual arrangement with her husband (who is also your patient) that allows each of them significant extramarital relationships, presents with a cough of 2 months' duration and dyspnoea on exertion. Physical examination reveals a regular tachycardia at 125, gallop rhythm, no murmurs, normotensive, raised JVP and hepatomegaly. Chest X-ray reveals evidence of pulmonary congestion. She asks you not to discuss her medical condition with her husband.

1. What is the most likely diagnosis and the initial management?
2. Extensive cardiological investigation later establishes a diagnosis: idiopathic congestive cardiomyopathy. Now what is the management?
3. You and the patient here face a rare and fatal illness, of unknown cause, with an uncertain natural history. What general principles of management do you establish?

P. R. Grantham, Vancouver

MR. CHARLES B.   AGED 48   FARMER   **330**

Charlie B., who seldom consults a doctor, presents complaining of increasing dyspnoea, which is impairing his capacity to work his dairy farm, which he manages with the help of his wife. He says this has 'crept up on him' over the last 2 or 3 years. He has smoked 30 cigarettes per day for the last 30 years and has a 'smoker's cough', mostly in the morning, when he coughs up about an egg cup full of clear sputum.

He is a thin, slightly-built man, with tanned, wrinkled skin. He looks older than his chronological age. He is breathless after walking into the room and for the first few minutes after sitting. He breathes through pursed lips. His colour is pink.

1. On this evidence, what diagnostic hypotheses would you be entertaining?
2. What further information would you seek?
3. What plan of action would you develop if your most probable hypothesis is verified?

W. E. Fabb, Melbourne

331   MISS D.R.   AGED 70   RETIRED SECRETARY

Miss R. has a long history of chronic obstructive pulmonary disease which has progressed to the point where she needs supplemental oxygen especially during exercise. She has been on prednisone 20 mg daily prior to admission to hospital and has steroid side effects including muscle weakness and osteoporosis.

1. How would you adjust her steroid dosage?
2. How would you treat her osteoporosis?
3. What other measures would be indicated in her rehabilitation programme?

C. T. Lamont, Ottawa

332   MR. J.A.   AGED 28   PLUMBER

At 2 a.m. you are called to see a male at home who cannot get his breath. He had been getting worse for the last hour or so. He was a plumber, aged 28 with no relevant past history. He had chest discomfort, some cough with frothy sputum and some wheeze. He had tachycardia, increase in jugular venous pressure, creps at both bases and some ankle oedema.

1. What disease process is occurring?
2. How would you manage the patient?
3. What is the prognosis?

E. J. H. North, Melbourne

MR. W.G.   AGED 72   RETIRED SHOPKEEPER   333

Fit and active with no past history of any significance, Mr. W.G. was seen during the night with an attack of acute pulmonary oedema. At that time his pulse appeared regular and he responded well to treatment.

When revisited the next morning he complained of palpitations and was found to be fibrillating (160 plus). Apart from fine basal creps there were no other abnormalities on examination.

Although home circumstances were good the GP thought that he needed admission to hospital for cardiac monitoring and treatment of his arrhythmia. He said as much to the anxious relatives then phoned the hospital to arrange a bed. Unfortunately the admitting physician did not feel the case warranted hospital care and advised digitalization at home.

1. What is the treatment of acute pulmonary oedema?
2. Was the decision to admit the patient a correct one?
3. What consequences are likely to flow from the refusal to admit and how can they best be coped with?

A. J. Moulds, Basildon, UK

MRS. N.   AGED 72   WIDOW   334

Mrs. N. who had a lifetime history of a heart murmur developed congestive heart failure 10 years prior to this time and had a diagnosis of idiopathic hypertrophic subaortic stenosis made by ultrasound 3 years previously. She had been on digitalis and diuretics for about 10 years. She presented complaining of acute shortness of breath, swelling in her ankles that had slowly developed over the preceding 1½ months and had reached the point where she was unable to walk more than half a block. There was no other contributory history.

The physical examination revealed a woman in left congestive heart failure. Diffuse rales were heard over both lung fields most marked at the base, with some oedema in her ankles. She was very careful about taking her digitalis and diuretics and on further questioning did mention that the pharmacist had substituted a new brand of digitalis about 3 months prior to this visit.

1. What causes of congestive heart failure must be ruled out in this woman?
2. Are different brands of drugs interchangeable?
3. What steps may be necessary because of variable bioavailability of drugs?

W. W. Rosser, Ottawa

TIMOTHY S.   AGED 9   335

Timothy had accompanied his parents to a Chinese restaurant with his sisters and brothers. During the meal he suddenly complained of difficulty with breathing. His lips and eyes had began to swell. The swelling of the lips had occurred 6 months previously, cause unknown.

He was brought to the doctor who made his diagnosis and treated him as an emergency.

1. What is the diagnosis?
2. What therapy was instituted?
3. What advice should be given to the parents?

B. M. Fehler, Johannesburg

336 MADAM P.L.H.   AGED 57

Madam P.L.H. a spinster has been under your care for the last year. Her main complaints are tightness of the throat, with poor appetite and weight loss. She also complains of associated flatulence and epigastric discomfort, and at times of sore throat.

Prior to seeing you she has had full investigations by a physician. Barium meal and follow through, oesophagoscopy, gastroscopy and blood tests were all normal. A tonsillectomy done by an ENT surgeon did not relieve her symptoms.

At the age of 35, she had a partial thyroidectomy for thyrotoxicosis. Last week you were called to her house because she developed difficulty in breathing. On arrival you notice hysterical over-breathing which settled with your management. You also noticed that she has been taking care of an aged, partially blind mother and obtained the history that she has been doing this for the past 10 years. In the last week her mother has been having frequency and dysuria and has been very demanding and difficult to manage.

1. To what extent has the house call helped you reappraise the diagnosis of your patient's complaints?
2. How would you now manage your patient?
3. How could your management of her mother's problems assist your patient?
4. What resources are available for the care of the elderly in your community?

F. E. H. Tan, Kuala Lumpur

337 MRS. F.B.   AGED 59   WIDOWED OFFICE WORKER

Mrs. F.B. complains of recurrent feelings of choking and difficulty in breathing accompanied by palpitations of the heart. The doctor notes a flush above the sternal ridge, extending into the supra-clavicular fossae and up the anterior surface of her neck. The symptoms have been present intermittently for 4 weeks.

1. What is your approach when there is a need to distinguish between the emotional and organic origin of symptoms?
2. If these symptoms prove to be emotional in origin what methods are available for Mrs. F.B.'s treatment?
3. What are your views on the label sometimes given to patients of 'suffering from mixed anxiety and depression'?

P. Freeling, London

MARION B.   AGED 15   SCHOLAR   **338**

You have known Marion for only about a year. She and her sister aged 16 have come to live with her mother whose first marriage broke up some years ago after which she married one of your patients 5 years ago. Marion had been living with her father and his new wife. She and her sister were unhappy and they decided to move in with their mother.

She comes in an anxious state because, for the past 3 days, she has been 'unable to get her breath'.

1. What questions do you ask her?
2. How do manage the situation?

J. Fry, Beckenham, UK

Wheezing

339 ROBERT S.   AGED 18 MONTHS

Robert was the second child in the family. His father was a carpenter, who suffered from asthma and they lived in their own home.

As an infant, Robert had atopic eczema which was now well controlled.

He had had no previous respiratory problems until 9 a.m. that morning when he developed a cough, wheeze and dyspnoea which had increased in severity over the following 2 hours, so that he was very breathless when mother brought him to the office.

1. What diagnostic possibilities would you consider?
2. What physical signs would suggest he had a serious disorder?
3. What treatment would you give him?
4. If he were not ill enough to require hospitalization, what advice would you give to the family?
5. How do you manage atopic eczema?

H. C. Watts, Perth, Australia

340 S.B.   AGED 3

Simon, an only child, has presented several times in the past 6 months with increasingly severe bouts of wheezing, lasting for several days, sometimes accompanied by fever and considerable malaise. Between attacks he is well but often has a muco-purulent nasal discharge. The parents, mother in particular, are very anxious.

1. What is the probable basis of Simon's condition?
2. What additional history might be of value?
3. What tests could be of value in diagnosis and treatment?
4. What would you tell the anxious parents?
5. How is treatment going to influence his condition?
6. What is the long-term prognosis and what is your long-term advice?

K. C. Nyman, Perth, Australia

341 MEHMET G.   AGED 10

Mehmet's family are Moslems; His father is a head waiter, and they live in a small, modern home. Despite ill health, his father manages to send both his sons to good private schools. Mehmet's brother has had asthma for years, but needs only occasional treatment. Now his mother brings Mehmet, saying that he has a cough and is breathless. You observe a slight wheeze on expiration, with some use of the accessory muscles of respiration. His mother is obviously concerned, although the patient is cheerful; she asks if this is asthma too.

1. What does the word 'asthma' mean to patient, mother and doctor?
2. How can further attacks be prevented?
3. Should this case be managed at home, or referred?

J. Grabinar, Bromley, UK

MARK A.   AGED 19   STUDENT   342

Mark, a well built athletic engineering student, complains that recently after training for sport or playing football, he cannot get enough air and feels quite distressed for some time afterwards. You examine him and find no abnormal signs.

1. What is the probable diagnosis?
2. What diagnostic tests could be helpful?
3. Having established your diagnosis, how would you treat Mark?
4. What are Mark's chances of eventual cure?

K. C. Nyman, Perth, Australia

KATHERINE J.   AGED 10   SCHOOLGIRL   343

This 10 year old girl, with a past history of asthma, is brought to you in the evening by her parents because they have been unable to control her asthma, which has been present all day. She uses a Ventolin (salbutamol) inhaler.
   The child is sitting up, has moderately severe bronchospasm, and appears anxious. The parents too look worried.

1. What are the possible causes of the child's condition?
2. What action would you take first?
3. What therapy would you consider? What are the indications for each form of therapy?

W. E. Fabb, Melbourne

MISS S.G.   AGED 14   SCHOOLGIRL   344

This girl is the eldest child of a large family. Her parents are separated with the mother caring for the children. She is a known asthmatic and her current therapy is Intal qid (for 4 months of the year), Ventolin inhaler 2 puffs qid p.r.n., Nuelin (theophylline) nocte. She has been well for the previous 4 months and you last saw her 2 months earlier when you reinstituted her Intal for the 'allergy season'. She presents to you one spring morning with an acute episode of asthma.

Examination reveals a pale girl with tachycardia and tachypnoea. She is using her accessory muscles of respiration and auscultation of her chest reveals high pitched inspiratory and expiratory rhonchi in all areas. She last used her Ventolin inhaler 3 hours earlier.

1. What are the possible aetiological factors in this attack?
2. What would be your short and long term management of this problem?
3. What is the significance of your examination findings?

D. S. Pedler, Adelaide

345 MRS. F. AGED 40 HOUSEWIFE

Mrs. F. has suffered from bronchial asthma for the past 2 to 3 years. Her condition has necessitated several admissions to hospital in the past, usually in 'status asthmaticus'. She is currently on prednisolone, 5 mg b.d. with salbutamol and beclomethasone by inhaler.

Mr. F. telephones at 6.30 requesting a home visit 'because the wife's a bit wheezy tonight'. He tentatively suggests a 'look-in tomorrow, when you're passing' will meet the situation.

1. In contacts with patients, family doctors usually accord some kind of priority in grading their responses: why do they do this?
2. What clinical phenomena constitute 'status asthmaticus'?
3. What might the doctor carry in his emergency bag to be ready to deal with this situation?

J. D. E. Knox, Dundee

346 JAMES P. AGED 15

James P. came when his usual doctor was on holiday, for a further prescription of his bronchodilator aerosol inhaler for asthma. It transpired that he had been wheezy most days intermittently for the last year or two – particularly in the morning, when it often woke him from sleep at 6 a.m. Other triggering factors were exercise and pollen sensitivity.

He was on no other drugs and his mother appeared to be unwilling to consider further therapy. The doctor detected an apparent general reluctance by both James and his mother to take his asthma seriously.

1. What would be the best way of assessing James' asthma?

2. How might the doctor handle the apparent unwillingness to take the asthma seriously?
3. What drug therapy might be considered for this patient?

J. C. Hasler, Oxford

MICHELLE V.   AGED 16   SCHOOLGIRL

347

Michelle has had bronchial asthma since early childhood when she was 'always in hospital'. Although she has coped better in her teens she has a perpetual wet cough and suffers from recurrent bouts of severe wheezing. Her effort tolerance is poor and, as a consequence, she plays very little sport. Her current medication is theophylline with salbutamol aerosol p.r.n. to relieve severe wheezing. On the advice of a friend, who is a patient at the practice, she seeks a second opinion.

1. What are the factors critical to the clinical assessment of this patient?
2. What factors will influence the doctor's management plan?
3. What are the important issues to be addressed in the education of this patient regarding long term management of her asthma?

W. L. Ogborne, Sydney

MRS. S.   AGED 70   PENSIONER

348

In your morning's mail is a note from Mrs. S., who writes: 'I would so much like for you to send me my sleeping pills and Ventolin inhaler. I have been very tired of late. I hear of a new drug to help my trouble – it's made by (pharmaceutical company): it's for all chest troubles. If possible, could I get this?'

You remember reading in the newspapers about a recently released antibiotic, hailed as a 'major breakthrough'. Mrs. S., aged 70, is house-bound, suffering from chronic obstructive airways disease, chronic bronchitis and emphysema, the latter of which is now the main impairment. You saw her last at home about a week ago, when she was depressed and complaining bitterly of her shortness of breath.

1. What are the pro's and con's of issuing prescriptions to patients without seeing them at the time of issue?
2. What is the role of antibiotics in 'secondary prevention', i.e. preventing exacerbations of chronic bronchitis?
3. Patients' needs are not synonymous with patients' demands. What factors govern the creation of patient expectations?

J. D. E. Knox, Dundee

349 MR. C.C.E.   AGED 28   UNEMPLOYED

Mr. C.C.E. is single. He has attended for 4 years and has suffered from asthma since childhood. He has a personality problem with low self esteem and confidence (certainly contributed to by his asthma) resulting in:

- – abuse of alcohol in the past.
- – current abuse of sympatheticomimetics (aerosol).
- – an inability to make friends (resulting in a tendency to promiscuity and several attacks of urethritis).
- – poor compliance.

He presents with a history of coughing up green-yellow sputum and insomnia. There is poor air entry, prolonged expiration and musical rhonchi all over. Pulse 120; physique good although somewhat overweight.

1. What determines someone's personality?
2. What constitutes patient compliance?
3. What prognostic factors are evident in this case?

D. Levet, Hobart

350 MR. H.D.   AGED 49   BUSINESS EXECUTIVE

This 49-year-old business executive with long-standing asthma arrived at the hospital with cough and fever of 2 weeks' duration. The illness, he tells you, began with fever, chills, cough, and muscle pain. Three days after the onset of his illness he was much improved, as was another member of his family with a similar illness. On the fourth day, however, when he awoke, he was sweating profusely and his cough became productive. His temperature rose to 103 °F.

1. What salient physical findings should be sought?
2. What laboratory aids might be expected to offer positive diagnostic information?
3. What are the most likely aetiological causes for secondary or post-influenzal pneumonia, more likely with underlying pulmonary disease such as asthma?

L. H. Amundson, Sioux Falls, SD, USA

351 MR. L.S.   AGED 62

This man's wheezing and breathlessness became worse and feeling that he had another chest infection he went to his doctor for antibiotics. For many years he had been subject to attacks of cough and breathlessness but recently the wheezing had become continuous and the breathlessness was now so marked that he was finding difficulty in keeping his job as an engineer. The doctor concluded that he had another chest infection and prescribed a course of tetracycline, 250 mg q.d.s. and Ventolin 4 mg q.d.s. The patient improved slightly but remained unable to return to work.

1. Does this patient suffer from bronchitis or asthma?
2. Discuss the management of late onset (intrinsic) asthma.

A. G. Strube, Crawley, UK

MRS. T.   AGED 23   BANK CLERK

352

Mrs. T. presented with a severe attack of bronchitis, her third in 6 months. There was marked accompanying bronchospasm. Initial response to treatment was poor, but eventually the symptoms subsided. On questioning, the patient admitted to smoking 40 cigarettes per day. Her peak expiratory flow on testing in the rooms was well below the normal range for her age and height. On being asked whether she felt she could give up smoking she replied that she had had a 'nervous breakdown' the last time she attempted to do so. She said she also gained a great deal of weight when she stopped smoking and that she had had nervous breakdowns on two other occasions.

1. Why was the patient's illness initially refractory to treatment?
2. How would you manage this patient further?

S. Levenstein, Cape Town

MR. L.B.   AGED 52

353

This man presented with a productive cough, wheezing and breathlessness. Three months previously he had suffered a myocardial infarct, but had apparently made a complete recovery and returned to work as a taxi driver. On examination there were signs in the chest and the doctor concluded that he had a chest infection and prescribed antibiotics and an expectorant cough mixture. Three days later another doctor was called in at night as Mr. B. was choking and could not get his breath due to the copious sputum he was coughing up. Again he had signs of congestion in the chest and the doctor concluded that the infection was resistant and so changed the antibiotic. As there was little improvement the patient came to the office and saw a third doctor who questioned him carefully about his symptoms: it seemed that although he was breathless on exertion in the day, with a tiresome cough and wheeze, it was not until night time that the breathing was really bad, when he was forced to sit upright in order to cough up the frothy sputum. If he lay down the difficulty in breathing became even worse. There was no chest pain. The doctor thought this sounded like the nocturnal dyspnoea of heart failure and with this in mind he examined the patient carefully. The pulse was 100 regular, blood pressure normal. There was some left ventricular enlargement but heart sounds were normal. Venous pressure was not raised and there was no ankle oedema: ECG showed the old posterior myocardial infarct. The chest X-ray report read: 'Extensive consolidation is present, particularly over the right lung field. A small effusion is demonstrated at the right base with bilateral enlargement of the heart.' He was admitted to hospital for treatment.

1. How could the diagnosis have been made earlier?
2. What is meant by the term 'congestion'?

A. G. Strube, Crawley, UK

Other respiratory problems

MR. G.   AGED 32   FARMER

354

A 32 year old single farmer had been seen by three physicians prior to seeing me. He presented with a history of fever, chills, cough, shortness of breath and generalized weakness. He had lost 25 pounds in the preceding 3 months. He had several physical examinations and diagnostic tests including sputum cultures, chest X-rays and four courses of antibiotics. He has been diagnosed as having recurrent influenza, acute bronchitis and chronic bronchitis. His condition was continuing to deteriorate.

On physical examination he was somewhat pale, and slightly febrile with a temperature of 38.5 °C. The only physical finding was a slightly elevated pulse rate of 90 and sharp crackling rales over both lung fields. There were no rhonchi heard in the lungs.

1. What further historical information is necessary to confirm the diagnosis?
2. What further investigations would be helpful at this point in time? Even though a chest X-ray was done one month previously would a repeat chest X-ray be of benefit?
3. Why have previous efforts to treat this man failed?

W. W. Rosser, Ottawa

MR. PETER Z.   AGED 57   STOREMAN

355

Mr. Z. was admitted to hospital with classical signs and symptoms of a right lower lobar pneumonia. This was confirmed on X-ray, and all other investigations fitted the diagnosis except that he was found to have a haemoglobin of 6 g/dl. He was treated with antibiotics and blood transfusion followed by parenteral iron and made a rapid recovery.

1. What investigations would assist in diagnosis?
2. If all your investigations regarding the cause of the anaemia were negative, how would you manage the patient in the future?

R. M. Meyer, Johannesburg

356 MRS. BETINA A. & MR. HARRY A. AGES: BETINA 42, HARRY 44
BETINA: HOUSEWIFE   HARRY: PANEL BEATER

You notice in your afternoon appointments that Betina and Harry A. have a joint appointment. You used to look after them 10 years ago when you were the doctor in a small rural community. You remember them as a pleasant, happy couple. Harry owned the local panel works.

Today they are coming about Harry's heavy head cold.

On meeting them you are struck by several things within the first minutes of the consultation.

- Harry looks physically unwell, with speech and breathing patterns that suggest he has obstructive lung disease.
- Both appear much older than their chronological age. This is particularly marked in Harry's case.
- Both appear to be unhappy, within themselves and with each other.

1. What are some common causes of accelerated biological ageing?
2. What diagnoses are you considering at this stage?
3. Given that you have limited time available, how will you manage the consultation from this point onwards?

M. W. Heffernan, Melbourne

357 MR. R.S.   AGED 38   TRUCK DRIVER

Mr. R.S. a 38 year old truck driver for a small bulk chemical company, was seen by his family physician complaining of a 3 day history of chills, cough, fatigue and lower abdominal pain. He was tender in the left lower quadrant, his lungs had left basilar creps and his chest X-ray demonstrated consolidation in that area. His white cell count was 6000 per cmm. Ten days later, he showed little improvement in spite of a course of antibiotics and his physician changed the antibiotic to erythromycin. R.S. improved slowly over the next 2 weeks and then returned to work.

Six months later, R.S. presented again to his physician with a similar complaint and reported that he had had one more episode between this and his last visit, which was similar, but of lesser intensity. On this occasion the patient mentioned that his wife had noted that these episodes seemed to come on each time he hauled nitric acid in his truck. Further questioning indicated that he filled his truck through an opening in the top of the tank and determined when it was full by watching through this opening.

The patient was referred to a respirologist with a special interest in occupational health, who confirmed the diagnosis.

The driver requested that his physician not report this case to the Workman's Compensation Board lest he lost his job. The chemical company was a small one, which was not required to pass government inspection and had no union, and the driver was due to be moved to an office job with the company.

1. What does the family physician suspect as the aetiology at the first visit?
2. How commonly do patients suffer from occupational related diseases?
3. What are the issues – ethical, moral and legal, relating to this man's concerns about reporting his disease?

C. A. Moore, Hamilton, Canada

CHAPTER 17

Chest Pain

This chapter begins with the diagnostic challenge of a series of cases of central chest pain in patients ranging from the adolescent through to the elderly. Then follow cases of right or left sided chest pain, a number of cases of actual or potential cardiac neurosis and some illustrations of work problems related to cardiac disease. Chest pain is one of the most common symptoms presenting to the family physician and often carries with it serious connotations. Patients often present fearing they have heart disease. The way in which the family physician manages these problems is of the utmost importance to the outcome. Failure to diagnose serious heart disease can result in the patient losing his life; failure to positively reassure the patient when no heart disease exists can result in the development of life-long disabling cardiac neurosis.

Central chest pain

358 **MR. B.P.   AGED 18   FARM LABOURER**

You have been asked as a rural practitioner to see a youth after hours with a story of having developed severe chest pains radiating to both shoulders and through to the back associated with sweating, shortness of breath and vomiting while playing football that day. It lasted about ½ hour and then recurred 4 hours later at rest. There had been several similar but less severe previous attacks over the last 6 months. There was no apparent relationship of the pain to respiration or posture. On examination he appeared pale, sweaty with an occasional irregular heartbeat and BP of 105/70; heart sounds normal; chest and lungs clinically clear.

1. What additional information is required to reach a diagnosis?
2. What possible causes should be considered?
3. How should this patient be managed?

T. D. Manthorpe, Port Lincoln, Australia

359 **JOE SMITH   AGED 33   ELECTRICIAN**

You know Joe Smith, although you haven't seen him as a patient for many years. He is known as the town's best electrician and is also very active as a coach with the local junior football team.

It's 1 p.m. Sunday and Joe has been brought in to see you because of an episode of central tight chest pain and headache which he developed at midday soon after getting up. The pain lasted about ½ hour, was associated with some light headedness and resolved spontaneously. There was no radiation and no other associated features. Until today he has generally felt well.

Last night Joe was out celebrating until 3 a.m. after the football grand final. He smokes 20–30 cigarettes per day and drinks on Saturday nights only. Over the last few years, he has been working 18 hours per day, 6 days per week because he says he needs to meet loan repayments and wants to 'get ahead'. All his clients want him to do the work (rather than his partner) and it's always urgent. He feels he has to oblige them. His wife and two children (aged 6 and 8) rarely see him and when they do he is cranky and irritable. This is beginning to worry him.

Physical examination is completely normal.

1. What are the possible causes of his chest pain?

38

2. What investigations are indicated?
3. What is this patient's main problem?
4. How would you manage this problem?

R. P. Strasser, Melbourne

MR. M.T.   AGED 31   CLERK

360

Whilst on call one evening you receive an urgent call to this patient because of an acute pain in the chest. On arrival you find him pale and hyperventilating, with incipient tetany. His wife is extremely anxious and upset.

Subsequent history and examination lead to the conclusion that the chest pain was caused by a muscle injury following lifting a heavy car battery.

1. What diagnostic possibilities would you consider whilst driving to the patient's home?
2. Why might he be hyperventilating?
3. What factors tend to make relatives particularly anxious about a patient's condition?

E. C. Gambrill, Crawley, UK

JOHN ROBERTS   AGED 48   COMPANY MANAGER

361

John, a visitor to your district, has been rushed in to see you by his cousin with whom he is staying. You notice John is pale, sweaty and tremulous. He tells you that 10 minutes ago he was sitting watching television when he noticed his heart thumping fast in his chest. After this he felt a tightness across the chest (no radiation) and a light headed feeling. He put an Anginine tablet under his tongue but it made no difference to his pain, although soon after he developed a thumping headache. The chest tightness subsides while you are talking with him.

Six months ago he had a similar episode and his doctor sent him into the local public hospital casualty department for a cardiograph. At the hospital, the doctors admitted him for observation, took blood tests several times and attached him to the cardiac monitor for 24 hours. He had returned to the hospital a week later for a test where he rode a bicycle. The doctors said all the tests were normal, but gave him the Anginine in case it happened again.

Apart from that one episode, John has no significant past history or family history. He mentions that his best friend and business colleague dropped dead last week from a heart attack.

Physical examination is essentially normal. ECG is within normal limits.

1. What is the problem in this case?

2. Are any further investigations indicated?
3. How would you manage this problem?

R. P. Strasser, Melbourne

362 MRS. S.S. AGED 45 CLERICAL WORKER

Mrs. S.S. had a hysterectomy for fibroids 5 years ago. Since then she has complained persistently of pain in the left iliac fossa. Laparoscopy, 3 years ago, showed a small ovarian cyst and this was later removed without relieving her pain. Sigmoidoscopy and barium enema were normal 1 year ago and neither the prescription of bran nor dicyclomine hydrochloride have relieved her pain. Mrs. S.S.'s father died 6 months ago and she remained severely depressed so that 4 weeks ago the doctor prescribed imipramine. You are called to see Mrs. S.S. in an emergency complaining of pains across her upper sternum, palpitations, and feeling cold and faint.

1. What is your differential diagnosis for the emergency consultation?
2. What is your problem list for Mrs. S.S.?
3. What are your criteria for giving antidepressant medication?

P. Freeling, London

363 MR. M.F. AGED 59 RETIRED CLERK

You receive a phone call at 6 a.m. from Mr. F's wife. M.F. is a very active man who retired because of moderate hypertension. Since his retirement his blood pressure has been well controlled on beta-blockers (140/90).

His wife, who sounds very worried on the phone, explains that her husband has had severe lower chest and upper abdominal pain for over one hour and that he is sweating profusely. When you see him shortly afterwards he is pale and very sweaty with a pulse of 90 and blood pressure 100/70. The remainder of the examination is normal. You perform an ECG which shows a pattern of a full thickness inferolateral infarct.

1. What are the aetiological factors in this man's myocardial infarction?
2. What is your management of this situation?

D. S. Pedler, Adelaide

364 HAROLD O'HALLORAN AGED 85 PENSIONER

The last time Harold was sick (3 years ago), he had pneumonia and your partner put him in hospital for intensive physiotherapy. In hospital he rapidly deteriorated becoming agitated and confused.

Today his daughter has brought him to see you because he was woken during the night by a severe central crushing chest pain that had lasted for about an hour. He says the pain was 'pretty bad' and he was very 'short winded' with it. His wife rubbed his chest with a hot ointment and eventually the pain went away. Harold says he wouldn't let his wife or his daughter call you because 'you young people need your sleep'. Physical examination reveals mild CCF and ECG shows signs of a recent inferior myocardial infarction.

Together with his 80 year old wife, Harold has lived in the same house for the last 30 years. His daughter and her family live next door. Apart from the bout of pneumonia, his general health has been pretty good, although Harold has been becoming more forgetful over the years.

1. How do you explain the episode of agitation and confusion three years ago?
2. Is hospital admission indicated this time?
3. Could you manage this patient at home?

R. P. Strasser, Melbourne

MR. M.S. AGED 42

365

Mr. M.S. was happily married with 3 young sons. He was a non-smoker who had been under considerable stress at work. He had a cold and a productive cough for the last 2 weeks and on the morning he presented, he had developed chest pain, a feeling of dull tightness across the lower chest, not related to respiration or exertion.

He was concerned that he might have heart disease as a colleague at work had had a heart attack 3 months ago.

1. What are the diagnostic possibilities you would consider?
2. What other information would you wish to obtain to arrive at a more precise diagnosis?
3. How do you exclude a diagnosis of ischaemic disease in a young man?
4. In a patient with proven ischaemic heart disease, when do you refer him to a consultant?

H. C. Watts, Perth, Australia

MR. K.W. AGED 38 BUSINESSMAN

366

Mr. W. presents with a history of central chest pain intermittently for the last 18 hours. He describes it as a burning tightness behind his sternum, it does not radiate, is not altered by food or liquids but seems a little worse with exercise. Pain began last night during intercourse, but at that stage it was not sufficiently severe to terminate the act, although the pain did keep him awake afterwards.

On examination he has a BP 140/95 (the same as on several previous occasions). The remainder of the examination is normal, as is the ECG. He has a family history of sudden death of his father aged 40 from heart attack, and his mother aged 51 from a CVA. He is known to have a slightly raised fasting serum cholesterol, about which he has done nothing despite advice. 18 months ago Mr. W. took over a neglected business, and with hard work, long hours and much worry he has built up a successful business. He smokes 40 cigarettes and drinks 4 whiskeys a day.

1. What is the significance of his chest pains?
2. What are the most important risk factors in cardiovascular disease?
3. What should you do about his other risk factors?

W. F. Glastonbury, Adelaide

367 MR. L.P. AGED 54 CLERGYMAN

Mr. L.P. presented with three episodes of substernal tightness over a 3 day period. One occurred after the exertion of gardening and lasted a few minutes. The second was related to tension at work and was also transient. The third appeared to be precipitated by a bout of coughing at bedtime and lasted intermittently all night. There was no radiation of the pain and there were no associated symptoms.

The patient is a non-smoker and physically active. He is married with three adult children. Six months previously he left an administrative job with the Church and took over as minister of a suburban congregation. There was a strong family history of coronary artery disease with the patient's father and several uncles all dying of this disease in their 60's.

The initial physical examination was normal. The cardiac rate was 74/minute and regular; blood pressure was 120/80. The initial electrocardiogram showed inverted T waves in the anterior chest leads V1–4 and two days later the ST segments were slightly depressed in the same leads. The electrocardiogram reverted to normal within a few days and there were no changes in the cardiac enzymes done serially over 4 days. The patient was treated with bed rest, nitroglycerine sublingually for the pain, isosorbide dinitrate and a beta-blocker.

1. How do you decide if chest pain is serious?
2. What diagnostic tests help?
3. What counselling do you give to the patient with coronary artery disease and to his family?

R. L. Perkin, Toronto

Lateral chest pain

MRS. C.D.   AGED 55   HOUSEWIFE

368

Mrs. C.D. presents with left anterior chest pain of recent onset. There is an unusual feeling in the skin associated with this pain. She has a past history of myocardial infarction and a left mastectomy for carcinoma of the breast. She smokes 20 cigarettes per day and has chronic bronchitis.

1. What is the cause of the pain?
2. What place have corticosteriods in the treatment of this patient?
3. How much of this patient's illness has been due to cigarette smoking?

B. H. Connor, Armidale, Australia

MR. A.W.   AGED 31   CLERK

369

Mr. A.W. complained of left parasternal pain which he first experienced carrying some heavy furniture when he moved into his new home with his wife and two children. The pain was at first acute and stabbing in character but it subsided to a persistent dull ache. A resting ECG was performed and found to be normal. An analgesic prescribed didn't prevent the recurrence of the stabbing pain when he again lifted heavy objects. A stress ECG revealed myocardial ischaemic changes.

1. How would you manage his clinical problem?
2. How do you prevent the patient from becoming a cardiac invalid?
3. How would his problem affect his family and his community?

F. E. H. Tan, Kuala Lumpur

WALTER M.   AGED 45   STOREMAN

370

Walter M. presented to his family doctor complaining of an acute right sided chest pain while lifting at work. He looked tired and pale and admitted to a loss of 13 kg weight over the past 6 to 8 weeks.

On examination his right chest cage was painful to pressure in the mid axillary line, suggesting rib fracture.

1. What diagnostic suspicions should these findings arouse in the doctor's mind?

2. What is the most likely cause of Walter M's rib fracture?
3. What matters should the family doctor discuss with the patient and his family?

W. L. Ogborne, Sydney

371 MR. T.S.   AGED 45   BUSINESS EXECUTIVE

Mr. T.S. had not attended the office for years. He was married with two grown-up children and held down a demanding job with a firm in the city. When he arrived to report his chest pain, he had just returned from a trip to Canada. He described a sharp localized pain on the right side of his chest. It was exacerbated by movement and inspiration. He admitted to smoking 20 cigarettes a day and to having a 'smoker's cough'. There was little to find on examination apart from some localized tenderness at the site of his pain, heavily nicotine-stained fingers and some bruising on his left upper arm which he attributed to horseplay with his young grandson.

A chest X-ray was arranged and showed two newly fractured ribs on the right and three healed rib fractures on the left. When Mr. S. returned for the X-ray results 2 days later he was at a loss to explain how the fractures might have occurred. On this occasion the doctor noticed a distinct smell of brandy on his patient's breath.

1. What is your differential diagnosis?
2. Which one diagnosis would most logically explain all the features of this patient's history and examination?
3. To what aspects of the history and examination would you pay particular attention in carrying out a routine check-up on a 45 year old man?

T. A. I. Bouchier Hayes, Camberley, UK

372 MISS P.C.   AGED 25   OFFICE CLEANER

Miss P.C., who works mainly in the evenings, consults you because of chest pain. She states she developed a cold about 10 days ago. A cough started 2 days ago, and she developed overnight a pain in the right side of her chest on deep breathing. She does not smoke. Her father, a heavy smoker, died of lung cancer. Your examination reveals a female, normal on physical examination, except for a slightly elevated temperature, and a friction rub audible at the site of her pain in her right chest. She can produce no sputum for examination.

1. What are the likely diagnoses here?
2. What investigations would you undertake?

3. Does a negative chest X-ray alter your diagnosis?
4. What is the significance of her statement that her father died from lung cancer?

D. U. Shepherd, Melbourne

MRS. J.P.   AGED 51   HOUSEWIFE

373

Mrs. J.P., the wife of a clergyman, still had two of her six children living at home. She was a cigarette smoker and worked part-time outside the home. She had head cold symptoms for 10 days which seemed to be getting better when she suddenly experienced over a 3 hour period chills and rigors, fever up to 39.5 °C, and a sharp pleuritic pain in the right lower chest posteriorly. She had a cough with purulent sputum but no blood or rusty sputum. There was a history of pneumonia on three previous occasions.

She was seen as an emergency on a house call. At that time she appeared acutely ill and had a friction rub over the right lower chest posteriorly and laterally with associated dullness and decreased air entry. She was immediately admitted to hospital where an X-ray showed consolidation of her right middle lobe. Her white cell count was 23,000. Sputum culture subsequently confirmed the diagnosis. Because she was allergic to penicillin, she was treated with erythromycin.

1. What is the pathogen?
2. How would you treat the patient?
3. What preventive measures would you advise for the future?

R. L. Perkin, Toronto

MR. B.F.   AGED 44   PLANT WORKER

374

This 44 year old male developed spontaneous chest pains which were associated with cough and dyspnoea but not with hemoptysis, vomiting, or wheezing. This recurrent chest pain had been occurring for 2 or 3 days with no previous history of chest pain. He had a history of hypertension for the past 8 years for which he had received intermittent oral therapy.

The history revealed one episode of thrombophlebitis of the left leg 3 years earlier; treated with bed rest, hot packs and stretch bandages. He was treated at home. The leg cleared in 7–10 days and he had suffered no recurrence.

Physical examination revealed a blood pressure of 160/110 and a pulse of 100. He was slightly dyspnoeic sitting in bed. Fundi showed grade I hypertensive changes, consisting of some arterial sheen and early AV nipping. The heart was slightly enlarged and a grade II systolic murmur was heard over the lower left sternal border. The extremities reveal 1 + peripheral oedema bilaterally. There was a negative Homan's sign.

1. What are the essential problems and their differential diagnosis?
2. What are the possible risk factors to be considered in this case?

L. H. Amundson, Sioux Falls, SD, USA

Other chest pain

MR. K.   AGED 45   BANK CLERK

375

Mr. K., currently being treated for hypertension with beta-blockers, saw the GP's partner just before he went on leave, complaining of chest pain. He was told that his pain was probably not of cardiac origin, but advised him to spend 3 days in bed and report back.

On coming to see the GP he said he had not had much pain over the past 3 days, but was clearly highly anxious. He wanted to know what the other doctor had thought the trouble was, and asked if he could go back to work. An ECG was performed which was normal. The patient was told this, and allowed to go back to work the next day. He was clearly much relieved. He was asked to return in a week's time for another BP check. His hypertension appeared to be adequately controlled.

1. What was the first GP's diagnosis?
2. Why was the patient so anxious at the consultation with the 'locum' GP?
3. Why was the patient relieved after the consultation with the 'locum' GP?

S. Levenstein, Cape Town

MR. C.H.   AGED 57   LABOURER

376

Mr. C.H., a skilled labourer, attended the office for the fifth time in 3 weeks. Once again he gave a graphic description of his chest pain which was sharp, situated just beneath the left nipple, unrelated to exercise and usually momentary. 'Do you think it could be my heart, doctor?' He was reassured, as he had been many times before, that the pain was nothing to do with his heart and that the tests which had been done had all been completely normal. Yes, he understood that, but still did not seem completely satisfied. The doctor checked his pulse and blood pressure. Mr. H. was not yet ready to leave the surgery. Despite being ½ hour behind time the doctor asked him to take off his jacket. He clamped his stethoscope over the site of the pain, listened intently and pronounced everything fine. Beaming broadly, Mr. H. left apparently happy.

1. What syndrome does Mr. H.'s story illustrate?
2. What are the reasons for frequent office attendance by a patient with no evidence of physical disease?
3. What resources are available for the health education of patients?

T. A. I. Bouchier Hayes, Camberley, UK

377   **MRS. S.H.**   **AGED 40**   **HOUSEWIFE/SOCIAL WORKER**

Mrs. S.H., a social worker by training and work experience, is a rather anxious happily married mother of three healthy children. She has presented six times in the past 3 to 4 years complaining of intermittent chest pain and numbness of her hands and has indicated each time that she is quite concerned that it is her heart. On each occasion she has appeared extremely distressed. Extensive investigation by the family physician and two different cardiologists has revealed no evidence of heart or other organic disease.

1. What investigations might be indicated at this most recent visit?
2. What referral(s) might be indicated at this most recent visit?
3. What is the most likely cause of this patient's symptoms?

G. G. Beazley, Winnipeg

378   **MR. J.P.**   **AGED 53**   **EXECUTIVE**

He complains of two pains:

One present for 2 months and located in the centre of the chest – quite severe and worse under stress – seems to be relieved by bringing up wind – may last 15–30 minutes – occurs several times a week – it feels tight and makes him feel rotten.

An upper abdominal discomfort which seems worse before meals and has woken him at 2 a.m. on several occasions. This has been present off and on for 2 years and is getting worse.

1. What would be your strategies for dealing with such an obviously complex problem in a busy consulting session?
2. How can you distinguish between the various causes of retro-sternal and epigastric pain?
3. What would you do if you're not sure of the diagnosis even if you have sought another opinion?

F. Mansfield, Perth, Australia

379   **LES B.**   **AGED 32**   **SALESMAN**

Les B. is a fit looking man recently discharged from the navy after 10 years of active service. He complains of aching discomfort in the anterior chest around the left breast often associated with a prickling sensation. He first noticed this in Singapore after loading 2000×50 lb artillery shells on his ship. Full investigations, including stress ECG, failed to reveal a cause at that time.

The chest pains and discomfort have recurred several times since but, despite numerous medical consultations and various tests, the problem persists undiagnosed.

1. What is the single most likely process by which Les B's symptoms will be diagnosed?
2. Why have so many doctors failed to diagnose the cause of Les B's chest pain?
3. During physical examination the spinous processes of T3 and T4 are very tender when firm pressure is applied with the thumb. What relationship, if any, does this finding have to Les B's chest pain?

W. L. Ogborne, Sydney

DESMOND K.   AGED 58   FACTORY MANAGER   380

This slightly obese patient with a history of attacks of gout presented 3 months ago complaining of transient retrosternal pain when playing the first hole of a round of golf. His blood pressure was 180/95 and the ECG was relatively normal. The pain responded to sublingual glyceryl trinitrate. He now complains that the pain has become much more troublesome over recent weeks. He has to take a tablet during his playing of every hole and he is experiencing pain when he takes his dog for a walk.

1. What are the characteristics of the pain of angina pectoris?
2. What action should the general practitioner take in relation to the patient's complaint at the most recent consultation?

J. G. P. Ryan, Brisbane

MR. M.N.   AGED 41   FORK HOIST DRIVER   381

Mr. N. consults Dr. Y. during Dr. Y.'s weekly visit to the factory. Dr. Y. is a GP in an industrial area, has many associations with industry, and attends clinics in two of the larger firms.

Mr. N. has been sent to the medical section by his foreman, who is concerned that Mr. N. seems to have had chest pain lifting some materials and on getting on and off the fork hoist. Mr. N.'s own doctor is thought to be treating him for obesity and anginal pain, and the foreman does not think Mr. N. should operate the fork hoist until Mr. N. has seen a specialist at the hospital outpatient clinic. Mr. N. is indeed overweight and has significant hypertension, despite the stated treatment regime. He is indignant about the foreman's attitude because he gets higher rates as a fork hoist driver, as well as better chances of overtime. His own doctor is overseas for two months and he refuses to visit the old doctor who is acting as locum tenens.

1. How should Dr. Y. advise the patient?

2. How should Dr. Y. advise the employer?
3. What should Dr. Y. do with regard to the patient's own doctor's locum?

P. L. Gibson, Auckland

382 THOMAS D. AGED 52 COMPANY EXECUTIVE

Thomas D. had been a senior executive with an important company but had been forced to retire owing to the development of angina and transient ischaemic attacks. Shortly before his consultation he had been informed that the Driving Licence Authority had informed him he was no longer eligible for a driving licence on medical grounds.

1. How would you manage the continuing care of his angina and transient ischaemic attacks?
2. How would you react to the decision preventing him from driving a car?
3. What responsibility does the general practitioner have in the prevention of arterial disease?

J. C. Hasler, Oxford

383 MR. W.R. AGED 65

Mr. R. had a coronary bypass operation at age 59 for intractable angina. He did well, requiring only chlorothiazide 0.5 g daily and propranolol 40 mg t.i.d. for treatment of mild hypertension (180/95 mmHg sitting).

At age 64 he developed intermittent claudication although his peripheral pulses were all palpable. This did not improve significantly when another beta-blocking drug was substituted, and withdrawal of this produced tachycardia. He was finally controlled on chlorothiazide and prazosin and is without adverse symptoms.

1. Are coronary disease and peripheral vascular disease related?
2. What is the basis for this patient's hypertension?
3. Is it rational to treat this patient's blood pressure?

A. L. A. Reid, Newcastle, Australia

Questions and Sub-questions

1. What clinical examination would you make and how would you do it?
    a. How would you endeavour to gain his confidence? Are there any special techniques in examining small children?
    b. What regions would you examine? If he were uncooperative, what would be the minimum physical examination you would perform?
    c. In what way, if any, does such an examination differ from that which a junior hospital doctor would perform?

2. What is the most likely diagnosis?

3. What predisposing conditions might be associated with this disorder?
    a. Do adenoids influence the onset?
    b. Is allergy a contributory factor?

4. What is the most likely causative organism?
    a. Is it likely to be purely viral or bacterial or both?
    b. If bacterial, what is the most likely organism?
    c. To what antibiotics is *Haemophilus influenzae* most sensitive?

5. What medications would you prescribe?
    a. What would you give for pain relief?
    b. Would you always prescribe antibiotics? If so, which one? If not, when would you see him again?
    c. Do ear drops help? What are their dangers?
    d. Are nose drops or decongestants indicated? If so, what would you use, for how long and how often?

6. What advice would you give the parents?
    a. When should they contact you again?
    b. Should children with otitis media always be seen for review?
    c. What should they do if perforation occurs?
    d. Are there any serious sequelae of such an infection?

H. C. Watts, Perth, Australia

290 M.N.   AGED 3

1. What are this child's problems?
    a. Does a clinically clear chest exclude the cough as a significant symptom?
    b. Is the past history of similar attacks of any significance?
    c. Could there be a problem present which is aggravating the otitis media?

2. What immediate treatment is indicated?
    a. Does the appearance of the drums modify the treatment in any way?
    b. Will drug therapy suffice?
    c. Is any immediate surgical intervention necessary?
    d. What type of antibiotic is indicated?

3. What advice would you offer to the parents about future management?
    a. When would you see the child again?
    b. What preventive treatment would you advise for the parents?
    c. Is referral for a specialist opinion justified and on what grounds?

T. D. Manthorpe, Port Lincoln, Australia

JOHN F.   AGED 6

291

1. What is the diagnosis?
   a. What are the causal organisms?
   b. What is the natural history?
   c. What complications?

2. What would you do?
   a. What regional examination would you do?
   b. Explain the disorder to mum?
   c. What treatment and why?
   d. What follow-up?

J. Fry, Beckenham, UK

DAVID M.   AGED 3

292

1. Why was the cause not recognized?
   a. The pain was unquestionably present in the cheek. What explanation can you offer for this?
   b. What clinical clues might lead one to suspect otitis media?

2. What treatment would you have recommended if the diagnosis had been made in the first instance?
   a. General measures?
   b. Specific treatment?

3. Do you regard otitis media as a medical emergency?
   a. If so, do you think a doctor should get up at night and visit a child whose parents suspect he is suffering from otitis media?
   b. What organisms are usually responsible for otitis media?

4. Would you wish to follow up the child?
   a. What is the prognosis of a perforated drum?
   b. What complications may ensue?
   c. Does a perforated drum have any late consequences with respect to career choice?
   d. How successful is tympanoplasty? Does the procedure have any late consequences?

J. G. Richards, Auckland

293 JAMES H.   AGED 7   SCHOOLBOY

1. What problems have occurred?
   a. Why is earache more prevalent on the right side?
   b. How could this problem be prevented?
   c. Why is the ear painful now following relief with discharge?

2. How would you manage this problem?
   a. What are the complications of otitis media?
   b. How would you diagnose mastoid disease?
   c. What complications may occur?

3. Discuss the infection process in this case?
   a. Should antibiotics be given for a viral illness?

E. J. H. North, Melbourne

294 MASTER J.R.   AGED 3

1. Is this just another attack of otitis media and 'bronchitis'?
   a. Does he have an underlying precipitating source of infection?
   b. Is each attack clearing completely?
   c. What other underlying diseases could be responsible?
   d. What investigations are indicated?

2. What do you want to know about the social situation?
   a. Are the parents able to afford adequate food, clothing, etc.?
   b. Is he being neglected by his parents, i.e. is this some form of child abuse?
   c. Are his parents giving him his medication correctly?

3. What long term effects are taking place?
   a. Is this permanently affecting his physical development?
   b. What are the effects on his physical development?
   c. Are these attacks in any way detrimental to the parent's marriage?
   d. What are the effects on the siblings?

W. F. Glastonbury, Adelaide

295 MRS. S.K.   AGED 29   SCHOOLTEACHER

1. How would you clarify this problem?
   a. Personal and family history?
   b. Physical examination?
   c. Office tests and investigations?
   d. Additional tests requiring referral?

2. What are the implications on the family, of a child suffering from permanent hearing impairment?
   a. Implications for the child?
   b. Implications for the parents?
   c. Implications for the other siblings?
   d. Implications for family function as a psychosocial unit?

3. What facilities in the community can assist the family to cope with a child suffering from impaired hearing?
   a. What is the role of the family physician?
   b. What are the roles of the practice nurse, health visitor, public health nurse, social worker and other health professionals?
   c. What specialized medical services are available in the community, and in the regional hospital?
   d. What facilities are available in the kindergarten and school?

4. Could Ronnie's hearing disorder have been diagnosed at an earlier age, or perhaps been prevented?
   a. What is the incidence of hearing disorders among children?
   b. What factors may contribute to delay in diagnosis?
   c. What children are at special risk for developing hearing disorders?
   d. What tests may be used for early diagnosis?
   e. What health education measures could assist in shortening the delay before diagnosis, or in preventing hearing impairment?
   f. Of what value is premarital counselling or ante-natal care in preventing congenital hearing defects?

M. R. Polliack, Tel-Aviv, Israel

MR. C.K.   AGED 50   ENGINEER   **296**

1. What measures do general practitioners take to enable patients, who are new to a practice, to make the best use of the services they have to offer?
   a. Under the National Health Service regulations, what constitutes a 'temporary resident'?
   b. What documentation is necessary to secure payment for a 'temporary resident'?
   c. What areas in Mr. C.K.'s life would it be appropriate to explore at the **first** consultation he has as a 'temporary resident'?

2. Deafness is a relatively common presenting symptom in family medicine. In general, what are common causes of bilateral deafness?
   a. What is the likely cause for Mr. C.K.'s deafness?
   b. What 'medical measures' might have been deployed in managing Mr. C.K.'s problem?

    c.   What might specialist referral achieve in Mr. C.K.'s case –
what is the specialist likely to do?

    d.   What degree of urgency should be accorded this referral?

    e.   What special risk might Mr. C.K. run were he to travel home by
air?

3.   Putting a patient on the 'sick list' is a common doctor activity.
Viewed in sociological terms, what does this activity entail?

    a.   What reasons might there be to justify the action in Mr. C.K.'s
case?

    b.   What details would the doctor enter on the sickness certificate?

J. D. E. Knox, Dundee

297   MR. G.   AGED 54   COMPANY DIRECTOR

1.   What advice will you give him related to his current infection?

    a.   What are possible problems if it is not settled prior to departure?

    b.   Will any treatment help?

    c.   Is there any place for antibiotics?

2.   What will you advise him about immunizations in general?

    a.   What immunizations are necessary?

    b.   Are immunizations effective?

    c.   How often do these require to be repeated?

3.   What is your advice about malaria prophylaxis?

    a.   Is prophylactic treatment necessary?

    b.   If so
       – when should it start?
       – how long should it be continued?
       – what would you prescribe?

J. R. Marshall, Adelaide

298   MR. GERALD M.   AGED 71   RETIRED SCHOOLTEACHER

1.   What are the likely contributing factors to his epistaxis?

    a.   How important is hypertension in epistaxis?

    b.   What changes occur in the blood vessels in the nose with age?

    c.   From where do most epistaxes originate?

2.   How would you manage this situation?

    a.   How do you estimate the amount of blood he has lost?

    b.   What immediate steps would you take?

    c.   What would you do about the blood clot in his nose?

    d.   How do you pack a nostril with an anterior bleeding point?

    e.   How do you pack a nostril with a posterior bleeding point?
    f.   What more radical measures are sometimes needed?

3.   What follow up will be needed?
    a.   If you pack the nostril, when would you remove the pack?
    b.   What advice would you give about preventing further epistaxes?
    c.   If the epistaxes recurred frequently, what would you do?

W. E. Fabb, Melbourne

G.P.   AGED 2½   **299**

1.   Why is the above history unsatisfactory?
    a.   In which bleeding diseases does family history offer useful information? His mother's brother had nosebleeds cured by cautery. Does this narrow the field of diagnosis?

2.   What would your next move be toward effective management?
    a.   What would be necessary to establish an accurate diagnosis?
    b.   What specific deficiency would enable you to diagnose Von Willebrand's disease?
    c.   How would you treat bleeding episodes?
    d.   Could you treat without admitting the child to hospital each time?
    e.   What problems might frequent hospital admissions pose, and for whom?
    f.   How could his trouble be readily identified by other doctors who might have to assume responsibility for him in an emergency?

3.   What are your intuitive feelings about this story?
    a.   Do you often see frequent severe episodes of bleeding in small children without demonstrable cause?
    b.   When are you as attending GP not reassured by other advice about your patient?

W. D. Jackson, Launceston, Australia

MR. C. CHAN   AGED 46   CHINESE RICE MERCHANT   **300**

1.   What further examination and investigations are required to establish a diagnosis?
    a.   What is the most significant sign or symptom in this condition?
    b.   What is the most significant predisposing factor so far known about this condition?
    c.   Does the fact that Mr. Chan is from the Chiu Chow Clan (a province of SE China) have any significance?
    d.   What office procedures can be performed by the GP to establish the diagnosis?

2. What is the treatment of choice?
   a. Is surgery indicated?
   b. Is there any place for radiotherapy?

3. What is the prognosis?

Footnote: Naso-pharyngeal carcinoma is particularly common amongst the Southern Chinese, especially of Chiu Chow origin. A predisposing factor in this condition is thought to be salt-fish ingestion.

N. C. L. Yuen, Hong Kong

301 MR. N.M. AGED 41 SAW MILLER

1. Is another referral advisable and if so, to whom?
   a. Is a full sensitization workup by an allergist indicated?
   b. How effective are desensitization courses in 'allergic sinusitis'?
   c. Could his occupation be relevant to this condition?

2. Do simple radical antrostomies have a high success rate in chronic sinusitis?
   a. This man originally had a nasal polypectomy. What does this suggest?
   b. The X-rays originally showed no abnormality in the sinuses. How does this result affect the overall management?
   c. Is the protection of the patient from over zealous procedural therapies a proper role of the GP?

3. Are there any simple measures that may be helpful?
   a. How can a doctor help a patient come to terms with his condition?
   b. Is simple saline douching of value in chronic recurring sinusitis?
   c. How effective are oral decongestants in contrast to local decongestants?

T. D. Manthorpe, Port Lincoln, Australia

302 MR. F.M. AGED 42 INSURANCE AGENT

1. What would constitute an appropriate differential diagnosis of this man's respiratory symptoms?
   a. What are the usual underlying causes of acute sinusitis?
   b. What are the potential pulmonary complications of upper respiratory infections?
   c. What are the usual complications of self-medication for nasal, sinus, and upper respiratory infections?

    d.   What is the differential diagnosis of mechanical interference with upper respiratory toilet?

2.   What are the ramifications of this man's heart murmur?
    a.   What is the importance regarding the need to accurately classify this murmur?
    b.   Would your recommendations for follow-up vary depending upon a diagnosis of rheumatic valvulitis, mitral valve prolapse syndrome, congenital defect, or functional murmur?
    c.   How important would antibiotic prophylaxis be in the event that a sinus problem required any manipulative treatment (such as antral irrigation or dental work)?

3.   What laboratory procedures would be of most value in assessing this patient's respiratory infection?
    a.   Can sinusitis be diagnosed by X-ray?
    b.   What would the likely sinus X-ray findings be if this represents acute maxillary sinusitis?
    c.   Would a culture of the mucopurulent nasal material provide the aetiological agent for this man's symptoms?
    d.   Would the finding on Gram stain and culture of the pneumococcus identify a likely aetiological agent?
    e.   What factors in the clinical course of this patient would dictate an ENT consultation for antral irrigation or a dental consultation for an infected focus in a maxillary molar?

4.   What are the expected outcomes of a general type screening examination, even for seemingly well-defined, localized problems such as upper respiratory infection?

L. H. Amundson, Sioux Falls, SD, USA

BETTY R.   AGED 2   **303**

1.   What was the most likely cause of her illness?
    a.   What other causes must you consider?
    b.   What complications might occur?
    c.   What treatment would you prescribe for this child?
    d.   How do you describe the probable clinical cause of the illness to the parents?

2.   If this condition were due to an infective agent, what other clinical manifestations could be produced by it?
    a.   What treatment is available for these?
    b.   What long-term effects might follow an infection by this agent?

J. G. P. Ryan, Brisbane

304 MR. Q.R.   AGED 65   RETIRED ENGINEER

1. What is the doctor thinking?
   a. Was the doctor careless when he first inspected the tongue?
   b. What percentage of ulcers of the tongue are malignant?
   c. How regular should re-inspection be in such a case?

2. What does he say next to the patient?
   a. Is it ever sufficient to make such a statement as 'Let me see it again if you are not happy about it.'? If so, does a doctor have to give definite instructions about what to look for? Or does he say, 'See me again in so many weeks.'?

3. What does he say to the patient's wife, whom he knows will be ringing up after the consultation?
   a. Does the doctor make conscious efforts to regain these patients' feelings of respect for his clinical ability?
   b. How does the doctor cope with all the uncertainties such a tragedy create in his mind about his clinical acumen? How can he reassure himself about the contribution of the patient, given that the patient was neglectful in allowing matters to proceed as far as they did before coming back?
   c. Was the doctor right to advocate by-pass surgery at 63?

P. L. Gibson, Auckland

305 DR. P.F.   AGED 32   UNIVERSITY LECTURER

1. How specific can a general practitioner be when diagnosing viral respiratory infections?
   a. What is the differential diagnosis of a tonsillar exudate?
   b. What place has antibiotic treatment in these cases?
   c. How rapidly do viral respiratory infections spread to other family members?
   d. Will the same infection present in different ways in other members of the family?

2. What viral infections cause concern during pregnancy?
   a. Is antibiotic treatment useful in any of these cases?
   b. Are any viral infections particularly serious in the last months of pregnancy or for the new born baby?
   c. In this situation, if the other children in the family become ill, should they be separated from the newborn baby?

3. How does a nuclear family cope when the only wage earner in the family is ill?
   a. What resources are available to help a family with young children when several members of the family are ill at the same time?

b. What advice should be given to a patient who is recovering from a viral illness but who is concerned about getting back to a busy job?

B. H. Connor, Armidale, Australia

S.P. AGED 5 **306**

1. What would be key diagnostic elements in the history and physical examination?
   a. Is the family history of siblings with a similar condition of any help?
   b. What is the significance of none of the children having had basic immunizations?
   c. What is the signficance of a friable white exudate covering the tonsils?
   d. What is the significance of tender cervical adenopathy?
   e. What is the significance of palatal petechiae?

2. What factors would be helpful in making a positive diagnosis?
   a. What is the accuracy of the aetiology of tonsillo-pharyngitis by physical findings alone?
   b. What are the advantages and disadvantages of the office use of the strep. plate?
   c. Would it be helpful to screen other family members for strepto-coccal carrier state?
   d. In view of the immunization status, should other culture techniques be utilized?
   e. If this patient has streptococcal pharyngitis, what are first and second line drugs used for therapy?

3. What other physical findings might help confirm or exclude a strep-tococcal tonsillo-pharyngitis?
   a. Bullous myringitis?
   b. Rhinitis?
   c. Hoarseness?
   d. Injected conjunctivae?
   e. Dry, hacking cough?
   f. Liver and spleen enlargement?

L. H. Amundson, Sioux Falls, SD, USA

TRACEY N.   AGED 4 **307**

1. How would you manage the present complaint?
   a. Would you take a throat swab and blood investigations – if so with what requests?

    b.   What antibiotic would you advise and for what length of time?
    c.   How would you promptly lower the temperature?
    d.   Is this a 'new' attack of tonsillitis?
    e.   What reasons underlie tonsillitis of such frequency?

2.   What advice would you give the parents?
    a.   In regard to possible tonsillectomy?
    b.   How to manage the hyperpyrexia and possible convulsion?

3.   Would you refer the patient to an ENT surgeon?
    a.   What history would make you refer patient to a surgeon?
    b.   What complications can arise from tonsillectomy?
    c.   What are indications for tonsillectomy?
    d.   How much is recurrent tonsillitis a compliance problem?

B. M. Fehler, Johannesburg

308   MASTER A.T.   AGED 8   SCHOOLBOY

1.   What immediate treatment is necessary?
    a.   Would you suggest an antipyretic?
    b.   Would observation suffice at present?

2.   When should antibiotics be prescribed in an otherwise healthy child?
    a.   If commenced, how long should antibiotics be continued?
    b.   Are antibiotics routine treatment for tonsillitis?

3.   What signs of complications would you look for?
    a.   What would you expect to find in the ears?
    b.   What would you expect to find in the chest?
    c.   What would you expect to find in the blood picture?
    d.   What would you expect to find in the urine?

4.   At this age, and with this history, what other diagnoses are likely?

5.   Is tonsillectomy indicated? If so, when?

D. U. Shepherd, Melbourne

309   DICK THOMSON   AGED 8   SCHOOLBOY

1.   Would you prescribe an antibiotic?
    a.   Are any laboratory investigations indicated?
    b.   Which organisms cause tonsillitis/pharyngitis?
    c.   Which antibiotic(s) would cover the likely bacterial causes of sore throat?

    d.   Which antibiotic is indicated in this case?

    e.   Even if this is a viral infection, why not prescribe an antibiotic?

2. Would you arrange a tonsillectomy?
    a.   What are the current indications for tonsillectomy?
    b.   Is a specialist opinion indicated?
    c.   What are the risks of tonsillectomy?

3. What other factors are there in managing this case?
    a.   What is Mrs. Thompson's understanding of Dick's illness?
    b.   How is the illness affecting Dick?
    c.   How will you deal with Mrs. Thompson's demand for a quick resolution of the illness?

R. P. Strasser, Melbourne

DAVID P.   AGED 10   SCHOOLBOY   **310**

1. What two problems face the doctor?
    a.   How would you cope with the father's anger?
    b.   At what stage of the consultation would you consider the father's anger?

2. What could be a differential diagnosis of David's condition given the few facts above?
    a.   Would you support your partner's diagnosis?
    b.   Would you suggest alternative diagnoses at this stage?
    c.   What would your treatment be?

F. Mansfield, Perth, Australia

MR. A.J.   AGED 25   UNIVERSITY STUDENT   **311**

1. What physical diagnoses would you consider to be likely?
    a.   To establish a working diagnosis in Mr. J.'s case, how extensive would you make your physical examination of Mr. J.? (i.e. out of the complete repertoire of 'the clinical examination', what items would you select as appropriate?)
    b.   What are the arguments for and against invoking laboratory assistance at this particular home consultation?

2. What problems, real or imaginary, may be inherent in this situation?
    a.   What special problems commonly face immigrants who fall ill in a 'foreign' country?
    b.   If, as seems possible, Mr. J. is suffering from an infection, in what ways might this influence the situation?

3. How would you manage this situation?
   a. What are the arguments for and against prescribing medicine for Mr. J.?
   b. What arrangements are commonly made for making available prescribed drugs during holidays?
   c. What follow-up arrangement (if any) would you make for Mr. J.?

J. D. E. Knox, Dundee

312   MASTER J.R.   AGED 6   SCHOOLBOY

1. Is it possible to determine the aetiological agent of an acute upper respiratory infection on the basis of your physical examination?
   a. Do you always do a throat swab for culture and sensitivity?
   b. When do you prescribe antibiotics, and if so, which antibiotics and for how long?
   c. When do you consider infectious mononucleosis in the differential diagnosis and what steps do you take to exclude this possibility?

2. What are the indications for tonsillectomy and adenoidectomy?
   a. Should all children have their tonsils out?
   b. Should any child have his tonsils out?
   c. Does frequency of acute attacks alone dictate the need for surgery?
   d. What is chronic tonsillitis and how do you make this diagnosis?
   e. How important is adenoid hypertrophy and how does it influence ear function, airway patency and facial appearance?

3. What is the role of allergy in the hypertrophy of tonsils and adenoids?
   a. Is size alone important?
   b. Why is it important to determine allergy before considering surgery?

R. L. Perkin, Toronto

313   MASTER Y.L.   AGED 4   ATTENDS NURSERY SCHOOL

1. What do you understand by the 'problem solving method', hypothesis forming', 'hypothesis testing', 'probability diagnosis', 'testing a hypothesis by treatment' and 'time as a diagnostic tool'?
   a. What are the most likely causes of this boy's sore throat, and what was the doctor's hypothesis?
   b. What is the predictive value of pus on the tonsils for a bacteriological infection?

c. If a bacteriological cause is isolated, which organism is it most likely to be?

d. How do you think a throat swab may have helped the doctor at the first and second consultations in hypothesis checking?

e. In what way did the doctor use time as a diagnostic tool?

f. Why was he waiting 10 days to re-check his hypothesis?

2. What are your indications for tonsillectomy?
   a. What are the disadvantages of tonsillectomy?
   b. Discuss the natural history/ies of tonsillitis in childhood.
   c. What condition/s has tonsillectomy been said to precipitate and why?
   d. How would you counsel the mother on tonsillectomy?
   e. If the doctor reacted angrily to the mother's suggestion, could his response have been appropriate?

3. Why did the doctor prescribe penicillin VK and for the length of time he did?
   a. Do you think the doctor should have stopped the penicillin VK after four days?
   b. Would he have been justified changing the antibiotic after four days with or without a throat swab?
   c. What might have happened had the doctor prescribed ampicillin/amoxycillin in this patient?
   d. In the highly unlikely event of this patient having diphtheria, how might the doctor's initial approach have affected the natural history of this disease?

J. H. Levenstein, Cape Town

MRS. J.A.   AGED 26   HOUSEWIFE   **314**

1. What is the likely nature of Dawn's problems?
   a. What do you understand by the catarrhal child syndrome?
   b. How would you treat frequent upper respiratory tract infections in a child?
   c. Discuss the advantages of adopting a practice policy for common conditions.

2. What are the indications for tonsillectomy?
   a. What is the relationship between social class and the incidence of tonsillectomy?
   b. What factors affect a patient's expectations of medical care?
   c. What resources are available to you to improve health education amongst your patients?

3. What are the possible reasons for aggression in a patient?

    a.   How do you deal with patient aggression directed against you?

    b.   What instructions do you give your receptionist about dealing with difficult patients?

    c.   What measures might you take if an irretrievable breakdown occurs in the doctor–patient relationship?

4.   What ethical principles govern relationships between medical practitioners?

    a.   What is your reaction when a patient criticises one of your partners?

    b.   How do you react when you feel that another doctor has undermined your relationship with a patient?

    c.   What steps can you take in your own area to avoid clashes over patient care?

T. A. I. Bouchier Hayes, Camberley, UK

315   MRS. FLORENCE A.   AGED 71   HOUSEWIFE

1.   How would you assess this patient?

    a.   What are the common sites for bones to lodge in the throat or oesophagus?

    b.   What importance has the history in impacted foreign body in the throat or oesophagus?

    c.   What are the usual features of foreign body in the upper oesophagus?

2.   How do you examine a patient with suspected foreign body in the throat?

    a.   How do you detect a bone in the pryiform fossa?

    b.   If you see no sign of the bone, what would lead you to refer the patient to an ENT surgeon?

    c.   How would he examine the patient for a possible foreign body in the oesophagus?

    d.   What radiological examination could be helpful?

3.   If the symptoms suggest a foreign body in the throat, but none can be detected, what would you do?

    a.   Could a minor laceration caused by the bone give similar symptoms?

    b.   If you decide to send the patient home, what advice would you give?

    c.   What follow up would you organize?

W. E. Fabb, Melbourne

KUMBURAI M.   AGED ?   TODDLER

316

1. What treatment should Kumburai have?
    a. What arguments are there for and against the treatment of acute upper respiratory tract infections with antibiotics?
    b. Should the mother's request for an injection be acceded to?
    c. What would she do if you said oral medication would be better?
    d. What good would a cough mixture do
        – for Kumburai?
        – for anyone with a cough?

2. Is Kumburai suffering from anything of extreme danger to him?
    a. What would happen to him if he should get gastro-enteritis, a lower respiratory infection or measles?
    b. If he had been breast fed, when would this have come to a sudden stop?
    c. What would Mrs. M. feel about future pregnancies if Kumburai should die?

3. What should Mrs. M. be told?
    a. On finding herself pregnant again, and believing that her milk was now poisonous to Kumburai what dangerous action might she take besides stopping the breast feeding?
    b. What beliefs might she hold about weaning foods?
    c. If Kumburai had been given an injection of procaine penicillin would her belief in injections as the only valuable therapy have been strengthened?

R. T. Mossop, Harare, Zimbabwe

JOHN W.   AGED 5   SCHOOLBOY

317

1. What are the likely causes of his condition?
    a. How would you distinguish between upper and lower respiratory tract infection?
    b. If there were no signs of respiratory tract infection and the rest of the examination was normal, what conditions might you suspect? What would you tell the parents when they ask, 'What's wrong with John?'?
    c. If in two days' time the child continues to have a high fever, but without additional physical signs, what conditions might you suspect?

2. How would you assess this child?
    a. What further history would you seek?
    b. What physical examination would you carry out, and in what sequence?
    c. What investigations may help in assessment?

3. What general advice would you give mother?
    a. If the child has signs of an upper respiratory infection, what advice would you give mother?
    b. What would you tell mother about fluid intake, food, rest and the use of antipyretics and tepid sponging?
    c. What follow up arrangements would you make?

W. E. Fabb, Melbourne

318   WILLIAM ANDREWS   AGED 2   INFANT

1. What possible diagnoses are you considering?
    a. Could this be a case of family problems presenting as sleep disturbance in the child?
    b. How does whooping cough present?
    c. What about nocturnal asthma?

2. What investigations would you do?
    a. What findings would you expect on chest X-ray?
    b. Would pulmonary function tests help?
    c. Is it worth allergy testing this patient?
    d. How about some blood tests?

3. How would you manage this problem?
    a. Is the mother's attitude relevant in management?
    b. What antibiotics are indicated?
    c. Which bronchodilator would you give and by what route?
    d. Would antihistamines help?

R. P. Strasser, Melbourne

319   MRS. O.R.   AGED 46   HOUSEWIFE

1. What is the diagnosis?
    a. Is 'acute chest infection with local moist sounds' specific enough?
    b. Would a patholological or aetiological classification of chest infection be of much practical value?

2. Is it either desirable or possible to determine the actual infecting agent?
    a. As *Streptococcus pneumoniae*, a virus or *Mycoplasma pneumoniae* are the likely causes and psittacosis, Legionnaire's disease and Q fever the unlikely ones, does sputum culture have anything to offer?

    b.   Will a pre-treatment chest X-ray be of value in diagnosis or in deciding therapy?

    c.   Is initial management the same whatever the cause?

3.   Which, if any, antibiotic is indicated?

    a.   What is the antibiotic of choice for a *Streptococcus pneumoniae* infection?

    b.   What two antibiotics could be used for a non-bacterial infection?

    c.   Should a broad spectrum antibiotic be used initially?

A. J. Moulds, Basildon, UK

E.P.   4 YEAR OLD GIRL   **320**

1.   What diagnostic hypotheses would be in your mind?

    a.   Could measles be a possibility?

    b.   Could the child be incubating measles having been immunized?

    c.   What other possibilities are there?

2.   How would you test your hypotheses?

    a.   What specific signs would make a diagnosis of morbilli?

3.   How would you manage the situation?

    a.   Is there any advantage in using antibiotics at the outset?

    b.   What are the common complications?

    c.   What are the less common complications?

4.   E.P. has a sister, aged eight months. Mother asks if you can prevent her getting the same condition. What would be your reply?

    a.   Is active immunization any use at this stage?

    b.   What is passive immunization?

    c.   Would it help in this case?

    d.   If so, when should it be given?

    e.   Will you need to actively immunize the baby later?

A. Himmelhoch, Sydney

MR. D.E.   AGED 18   COLLEGE STUDENT   **321**

1.   Is your first diagnosis correct?

    a.   What is the normal course of influenza?

    b.   Is there any advantage in using antibiotics at the first visit?

2.   On the second visit, what do you think has happened?

    a.   Could he die? If so, from what?

    b.   Before using antibiotics, should you consider doing any pathology tests?

    c.   Does the fact that he played football have any bearing on the course this illness may take?

    d.   What is the most lethal bacterium which can colonize as secondary infection in influenza?

    e.   Can the influenza virus cause death without secondary bacterial infection?

A. Himmelhoch, Sydney

322   DEREK B.   AGED 40   CIVIL SERVANT

1. What are the main diagnoses that you would consider for this pyrexial episode?
    a. How significant is a holiday in the Mediterranean?
    b. Is the general practitioner's list of differential diagnoses likely to be different from the specialist's?

2. What investigations might you order?
    a. What investigations are likely to give you the biggest yield?
    b. What factors influence the point at which the general practitioner starts to order investigations?
    c. What are the chances all your investigations will be negative?

3. How does a patient's past history influence the doctor's approach and management?
    a. Is a doctor prejudiced in his approach and management to a patient with frequent psychological and emotional problems?
    b. What effect might anxiety have on the presentation of physical illness?

J. C. Hasler, Oxford

323   MR. D.C.   AGED 40   COMPANY EXECUTIVE

1. Should you discuss his obvious embarrassment?
    a. Should you tell him to 'be a man' and ignore minor inconveniences?
    b. Should you tell him to 'stand up to his wife'?
    c. Should you concentrate on his physical symptom?

2. What are the likely physical findings in this case?
    a. Which systems in particular would be examined?
    b. Is a physical examination necessary?

3. If the physical findings are negative, should a chest X-ray be performed?
   a. What other investigations are mandatory?

4. Should the management include a cough suppressant?
   a. Should management of this problem include anything other than pharmaceutical prescriptions?

D. U. Shepherd, Melbourne

MR. A.C.   AGED 32   STOREMAN   **324**

1. If your physical examination indicates no specific abnormal findings, with the exception of possible weight loss, what are the most likely diagnoses?

2. What investigations are indicated in this case?
   a. What would you be looking for in a chest X-ray?
   b. Should the pharynx be carefully examined?
   c. Would X-ray of the nasal sinuses be of help in this case?
   d. Could examination of sputum be of help?
   e. Is bronchoscopy indicated?

3. What would you prescribe for this cough?
   a. If no carcinoma of the lung is found?
   b. If a carcinoma is found?

4. If the cough proves to be simply related to excessive smoking, how would you handle this problem?

D. U. Shepherd, Melbourne

MR. JOHN J.   AGED 75   **325**

1. Why should the doctor arrange a chest X-ray?
   a. What are the likely differential diagnoses?
   b. Do any of them matter at the age of 75?

2. The chest X-ray showed a carcinoma of the bronchus. What would be the doctor's immedite course of action?
   a. What treatment is available?
   b. Is it effective?

3. The chest specialist recommended no treatment. How would the doctor manage the case now?
   a. What would he say to the patient?
   b. What would he say to his wife?

J. C. Hasler, Oxford

326   THOMAS R.   AGED 62

1. What are the long term complications of partial gastrectomy?
   a. What follow-up would you organize for such patients in your practice?
   b. How would you check on non-compliers?
   c. What investigations would you arrange, why and how often?

2. Give your assessment of his new symptoms.
   a. What would you do at this consultation?
   b. What explanation would you give T.R.?

3. How would you manage the likely conditions that you discover?
   a. How do you treat post-gastrectomy anaemia?
   b. What is the prognosis of the angina in T.R.?

J. Fry, Beckenham, UK

327   MR. & MRS. S.   AGED 64 AND 62   PENSIONERS

1. What was the best way of managing Mrs. S.?
   a. Was the GP justified in regarding her symptoms as psycho-somatic?
   b. Were investigations necessary to establish the psychogenicity of her symptoms?
   c. Why do patients sometimes persist with irrational fears about their physical health?
   d. Can phobias about illness sometimes mask other problems in the patient's life?
   e. How should the GP go about trying to discover what might be troubling Mrs. S.?
   f. What approach should he adopt if she persists in saying that there is nothing troubling her?
   g. Should psychotropic drugs have been used on Mrs. S.?
   h. Should further investigations have been performed if Mrs. S. had refused to accept the negative findings of the tests the GP had arranged?
   i. Should Mrs. S. have been offered specialist referral if she had refused to accept the GP's assurance about her physical health?

2. What was the cause of Mr. S.'s symptoms?
   a. What is the likeliest cause of gastro-intestinal bleeding in this patient?
   b. How great are the chances of a malignancy being found?

3. Was there any connection between Mrs. S.'s symptoms and those of her husband?

a. To what extent can marital difficulties cause psychosomatic symptoms?
b. To what extent could Mrs. S.'s mental state have contributed to the development of an ulcer in her husband?
c. What role do psychogenic factors play in the development and activity of peptic ulcers?
d. If the ulcer is found to be malignant, would this lead you to think that psychogenic factors did not play a significant part in its causation?

4. How are Mr. and Mrs. S. likely to present in the future?
   a. Can an increase in Mrs. S.'s symptoms be expected?
   b. How is the relationship between Mr. and Mrs. S. likely to be affected by his illness?
   c. How should the GP manage the medical and psychological problems which can be expected to arise in this couple?

S. Levenstein, Cape Town

MR. J.G.   AGED 76   **328**

1. Should surgery be performed?
   a. Is it reasonable to think of withholding surgery?
   b. Do you have a right to withhold it?
   c. What sort of surgery might be done?

2. Would you discuss the whole problem with the patient?
   a. What might your reasons be for frankly discussing the situation with your patient?
   b. How do you handle his son's request not to tell Dad the diagnosis?
   c. How can you proffer options to this man?

3. How could he be offered the best hope for successful surgery if that is the chosen option?
   a. What preparation will be required remembering that he has been taking aminophylline, prednisolone, and a diuretic?
   b. Would you avoid any particular drugs – why?
   c. Any particular dangers in the postoperative period?

W. D. Jackson, Launceston, Australia

MRS. I.S.   AGED 45   **329**

1. What is the most likely diagnosis and the initial management?
   a. What tests might you order yourself before prescribing any treatment?

b. Do you initiate pharmacotherapy before a cardiological consultation?
c. Is dietary manipulation indicated?
d. Is her lifestyle a problem for you?

2. Extensive cardiological investigation later establishes a diagnosis: idiopathic congestive cardiomyopathy. Now what is the management?
   a. What is the long term prognosis?
   b. What are the complications of long term therapy for this condition?
   c. Can she be managed at home or will hospital be necessary?

3. You and the patient here face a rare and fatal illness, of unknown cause, with an uncertain natural history. What general principles of management do you establish?
   a. How do you describe the prognosis to the patient?
   b. Should you discuss the expected course and prognosis with her husband?
   c. When and how do you approach terminal parental illness with children?

P. R. Grantham, Vancouver

330 MR. CHARLES B.   AGED 48   FARMER

1. On this evidence, what diagnostic hypotheses would you be entertaining?
   a. What are the clinical characteristics of chronic obstructive lung disease?
   b. What is the distinction between the so called 'pink puffer' and the 'blue bloater'?
   c. What are the pathological elements which constitute chronic obstructive lung disease?

2. What further information would you seek?
   a. What past history is important?
   b. What features would you look for on physical examination?
   c. What investigations would give useful information?

3. What plan of action would you develop if your most probable hypothesis is verified?
   a. What regime would you initiate for this case of chronic obstructive lung disease in a self-employed farmer?
   b. What preventive measures would you advise?
   c. How would you help Mr. B. to use health care resources more appropriately in the future?

d.   What would you tell Mr. B. about his condition, what you intend to do about it, what he should do about it, and his long-term outlook?

W. E. Fabb, Melbourne

MISS D.R.   AGED 70   RETIRED SECRETARY   **331**

1.   How would you adjust her steroid dosage?
   a.   Alternate day dosage or continuous?
   b.   Outline a suitable dose reduction regime.

2.   How would you treat her osteoporosis?
   a.   Would you recommend oestrogen therapy?
   b.   What other medications or supplements? What dosage?

3.   What other measures would be indicated in her rehabilitation programme?
   a.   Portable oxygen?
   b.   Physiotherapy?
   c.   Other measures?

C. T. Lamont, Ottawa

MR. J.A.   AGED 28   PLUMBER   **332**

1.   What disease process is occurring?
   a.   What tests would you perform in the home to possibly diagnose this case?
   b.   His urine test had heavy proteinuria and showed traces of blood – Why?
   c.   What further tests might be undertaken?
   d.   What are the causes of CCF?
   e.   What other information should be sought?

2.   How would you manage the patient?
   a.   In the short term?
   b.   In the long term?

3.   What is the prognosis?
   a.   Is it likely to recur?
   b.   Is long term therapy of use?
   c.   How long should this be undertaken?

E. J. H. North, Melbourne

333 MR. W.G.   AGED 72   RETIRED SHOPKEEPER

1. What is the treatment of acute pulmonary oedema?
    a. Is there any useful advice that can be given on the phone before the doctor sets out to see the patient?
    b. Is oxygen essential, desirable or not necessary at home?
    c. What drugs/dosages/routes of administration should be used?

2. Was the decision to admit the patient a correct one?
    a. Has a 'silent' infarct been excluded?
    b. Will cardiac monitoring improve his chances of survival?
    c. If the GP had an ECG machine and/or a portable defibrillator would that make home care more feasible?
    d. Can the relatives realistically be expected to cope?
    e. Can the GP realistically be expected to cope?

3. What consequences are likely to flow from the refusal to admit and how can they best be coped with?
    a. Will the relatives now think the GP does not know what he is doing?
    b. Should the GP call an ambulance and send the patient anyway?
    c. If he decides to treat the patient at home what instructions should be given to the relatives?
    d. If the patient dies during the night who is going to look silly – the GP or the hospital physician?

A. J. Moulds, Basildon, UK

334 MRS. N.   AGED 72   WIDOW

1. What causes of congestive heart failure must be ruled out in this woman?
    a. What are the most common causes of congestive heart failure?
    b. What role could this woman's social circumstances play in the development of congestive heart failure?
    c. Could the drug change have had any impact?

2. Are different brands of drugs interchangeable?
    a. What factors influence the bioavailability of the drug?
    b. Can bioavailability be accurately tested?
    c. Is bioavailability of drugs more important in some drugs than others?

3. What steps may be necessary because of variable bioavailability of drugs?
    a. Name drugs in which there is variable bioavailability.

b. How may physicians avoid the above situation?

c. What role does the patient's health play in bioavailability?

W. W. Rosser, Ottawa

TIMOTHY S.   AGED 9   **335**

1. What is the diagnosis?
   a. Is this an acute allergic reaction due to an unknown allergen?
   b. How dangerous is the outcome if left untreated?
   c. How certain can you be of your diagnosis?

2. What therapy was instituted?
   a. Is the use of cortisone indicated?
   b. Should we use adrenaline subcutaneously?
   c. Are antihistamines of value?
   d. Is hospitalization necessary?

3. What advice should be given to the parents?
   a. What tests are available to discover the allergen?
   b. Is desensitizing of benefit to the child?
   c. Should parents be informed in the use of an emergency kit of cortisone and antihistamines and adrenaline?
   d. What dangers can possibly occur with the child?

B. M. Fehler, Johannesburg

MADAM P.L.H.   AGED 57   **336**

1. To what extent has the house call helped you reappraise the diagnosis of your patient's complaints?
   a. Discuss the differential diagnosis of dysphagia?
   b. What is 'globus hystericus'? To what extent are you now able to label your patient's complaints as functional?
   c. What is the place of endoscopy in this patient?

2. How would you now manage your patient?
   a. Define 'empathy'. How would this attitude assist your patient?
   b. If you inform the patient that her symptoms are functional, do you then discharge her from your care?
   c. What is the most likely prognosis for your patient?

3. How could your management of her mother's problems assist your patient?
   a. What are the clinical features of cataract?
   b. How would you rule out the possibility of diabetes in her mother?

    c.   How could you mobilize help from members of the family to assist your patient?

4.   What resources are available for the care of the elderly in your community?
    a.   Discuss the 'pros' and 'cons' of admitting your patient's mother to an institution.

F. E. H. Tan, Kuala Lumpur

337   MRS. F.B.   AGED 59   WIDOWED OFFICE WORKER

1.   What is your approach when there is a need to distinguish between the emotional and organic origin of symptoms?
    a.   Would the probabilities of differential diagnoses be changed if Mrs. F.B. was a male?
    b.   What do you understand patients to mean when they say they have palpitations? How do you clarify their meaning with them?

2.   If these symptoms prove to be emotional in origin what methods are available for Mrs. F.B.'s treatment?
    a.   What are the differences between 'operant' and 'Pavlovian' conditioning?
    b.   What are the associated symptoms of hyperventilation and what is their physical explanation?
    c.   On what other occasions may people voluntarily hyperventilate? Are there risks in doing so?

3.   What are your views on the label, sometimes given to patients, of 'suffering from mixed anxiety and depression'?
    a.   What are the pros and cons of giving benzodiazepines for symptoms of anxiety apparently produced by recent stress?
    b.   Are there any effects on mortality of the recent loss of a spouse? If there are, are they uniform for both genders? How might they be explained?

P. Freeling, London

338   MARION B.   AGED 15   SCHOLAR

1.   What questions do you ask her?
    a.   What conditions do you consider in order of frequency?
    b.   What do you expect to find on examining her?

2.   How do you manage the situation?
    a.   What do you tell Marion?

b.   What treatment do you give her?
c.   What is the prognosis of the syndrome?

J. Fry, Beckenham, UK

ROBERT S.   AGED 18 MONTHS   **339**

1.   What diagnostic possibilities would you consider?
   a.   What signs would suggest a diagnosis of asthma?
   b.   What would make you consider a foreign body?
   c.   Could he have bronchiolitis?
   d.   What other diagnostic possibilities should be considered?

2.   What physical signs would suggest he had a serious disorder?
   a.   Colour?
   b.   Respiratory rate?
   c.   Pulse rate and character?
   d.   Ability to take fluids?

3.   What treatment would you give him?
   a.   Are any medications effective for asthma in a child this age?
   b.   Is inability to drink fluids a serious sign? Why?

4.   If he were not ill enough to require hospitalization, what advice
     would you give to the family?
   a.   What signs should alert them to seek review?
   b.   How much fluid should he take?
   c.   Would you tell the parents he had 'asthma'?
   d.   What possible allergic factors should be considered?

5.   How do you manage atopic eczema?
   a.   What local therapy?
   b.   Do oral medications help?
   c.   Does diet have a role in aggravating eczema?

H. C. Watts, Perth, Australia

S.B.   AGED 3   **340**

1.   What is the probable basis of Simon's condition?
   a.   Discuss the allergic diathesis.
   b.   How much does infection have a role?
   c.   Is it usual to find a specific allergen in such a case?

2.   What additional history might be of value?
   a.   Would you expect a history of skin problems or food allergies in
        infancy?

    b.   What related conditions could occur in his family history?

    c.   What specific enquiries about Simon's environment would you make?

3.   What tests could be of value in diagnosis and treatment?
    a.   Discuss the role of skin testing and the RAST test for allergies.
    b.   Is there a place for empiric testing – e.g., a trial of removal of all milk products for a short period?

4.   What would you tell the anxious parents?
    a.   Explain the allergic process in lay terms?
    b.   What changes in environment would you recommend, if any?
    c.   Would you advise a normal life-style for Simon?

5.   How is treatment going to influence his condition?
    a.   How and when would antibiotics be used?
    b.   What other therapies are useful?
    c.   Would you consider Simon a candidate for 'Interval Therapy'?
    d.   Which activities should be specifically encouraged?

6.   What is the long-term prognosis and what is your long-term advice?
    a.   Is the condition likely to persist into adolescence?
    b.   What would you advise the parents about Simon's activities?
    c.   The parents are worried about the same problem developing in any other children they might have. How would you counsel them?

K. C. Nyman, Perth, Australia

341   MEHMET G.   AGED 10

1.   What does the word 'asthma' mean to patient, mother and doctor?
    a.   What is the difference between asthma and bronchitis in children?
    b.   How can you establish the reversibility of airways obstruction?
    c.   What signs and tests give a good idea of the progress of the disease?

2.   How can further attacks be prevented?
    a.   What roles do infection, allergy, exercise and stress play?
    b.   What prophylactic measures can be used?
    c.   What prognosis can you give mother?
    d.   What forms of exercise are beneficial?

3.   Should this case be managed at home, or referred?
    a.   When is asthma dangerous?

b. What emergency treatment can be given in a severe attack?
c. When, if ever, should the patient be separated from his parents?

J. Grabinar, Bromley, UK

MARK A.　AGED 19　STUDENT　　　342

1. What is the probable diagnosis?
    a. What pointers might there be in Mark's past history?
    b. Could the family history be helpful?

2. What diagnostic tests could be helpful?
    a. Discuss the use of ventilatory function tests for such patients.
    b. What is the place of blood tests and chest X-ray in Mark's case?
    c. Would you consider a trial of empirical therapy?

3. Having established your diagnosis, how would you treat Mark?
    a. What is the place of cromoglycate?
    b. How would you use bronchodilators in this case?
    c. Would you use allergy testing, and if so what would you expect
        to achieve?

4. What are Mark's chances of eventual cure?
    a. Is his condition likely to be life-long?
    b. Would you advise against sport?
    c. Is his condition likely to worsen?

K. C. Nyman, Perth, Australia

KATHERINE J.　AGED 10　SCHOOLGIRL　　　343

1. What are the possible causes of the child's condition?
    a. Could Katherine's condition be due to inadequate or incorrect
        use of her medication?
    b. What role does respiratory infection play in resistant asthma?
    c. What emotional factors operate in such cases?

2. What action would you take first?
    a. How would you assess the child's condition?
    b. Does chest radiology provide useful additional information in
        such cases?
    c. What value are respiratory function tests under these
        circumstances?

3. What therapy would you consider? What are the indications for each
    form of therapy?
    a. With what specific therapy would you begin, and why?

b.   What would be your second line of treatment if the first failed, and why?

c.   Under what circumstances would you consider hospital admission?

d.   If you send the patient home, what advice would you give the parents?

e.   What opportunity does this situation present for preventive care and health promotion?

f.   What follow up would you arrange?

W. E. Fabb, Melbourne

344   MISS S.G.   AGED 14   SCHOOLGIRL

1.   What are the possible aetiological factors in this attack?
   a.   What is the significance of the family situation?
   b.   What is the significance of the time of the year?
   c.   What would you expect to be the compliance of this girl with her current therapy?

2.   What would be your short and long term management of this problem?
   a.   What is the role of nebulized Ventolin?
   b.   What is the value of Intal in an acute attack?
   c.   Does the occurrence of this attack alter your long term management?

3.   What is the significance of your examination findings?
   a.   The lack of an obvious precipitating cause?
   b.   The pallor?
   c.   What effect does a chronic disease have on growth?
   d.   In the presence of markedly decreased air entry, how accurate an assessment of lung function can you obtain with a stethoscope?

D. S. Pedler, Adelaide

345   MRS. F.   AGED 40   HOUSEWIFE

1.   In contacts with patients, family doctors usually accord some kind of priority in grading their responses: why do they do this?
   a.   What questions might the doctor ask Mr. F. to clarify the issue of degree or urgency?

2.   What clinical phenomena constitute 'status asthmaticus'?
   a.   If the doctor finds Mrs. F. in status, does the fact that she is already taking prednisolone by mouth influence management?

3. What might the doctor carry in his emergency bag to be ready to deal with this situation?
   a. How do doctors cope with the need to comply with security regulations and also ensure ready availability of potent drugs?

J. D. E. Knox, Dundee

JAMES P.   AGED 15   346

1. What would be the best way of assessing James' asthma?
   a. What are the common patterns of asthma in relation to triggering factors and time of day?
   b. Why can patients have quite severe asthma and yet produce normal peak expiratory flow rates in the middle of the morning?
   c. What place does a peak flow meter have in the assessment of asthma?

2. How might the doctor handle the apparent unwillingness to take the asthma seriously?
   a. What are the likely reasons for this attitude?
   b. What specific approaches in the consultation are likely to be productive or otherwise?

3. What drug therapy might be considered for this patient?
   a. What are the advantages and disadvantages of aerosols versus oral medication?

J. C. Hasler, Oxford

MICHELLE V.   AGED 16   SCHOOLGIRL   347

1. What are the factors critical to the clinical assessment of this patient?
   a. What information should be sought in taking the history?
   b. What information should be sought in the physical examination?
   c. What investigation should be performed in order to define the nature and severity of Michelle's disability?

2. What factors will influence the doctor's management plan?
   a. What is the value of skin tests for allergens?
   b. What tests can or should be performed in the consulting room to assess Michelle's response to bronchodilators?
   c. How might beta stimulator aerosols be used more effectively with this patient?
   d. What other drug therapies are likely to be beneficial and how is this best evaluated?

3. What are the important issues to be addressed in the education of this patient regarding long term management of her asthma?
   a. What special advice should be given concerning respiratory tract infection?
   b. What special advice should be given regarding the use of aerosols?
   c. How can the doctor and the patient ensure that continuity of medical care is guaranteed despite the problems of holidays, travel and communications?

W. L. Ogborne, Sydney

348 MRS. S.   AGED 70   PENSIONER

1. What are the pro's and con's of issuing prescriptions to patients without seeing them at the time of issue?
   a. What systems exist for regulating 'repeat prescriptions'?
   b. What are the basic features of a repeat prescription card, which many practices now use?

2. What is the role of antibiotics in 'secondary prevention', i.e. preventing exacerbations of chronic bronchitis?
   a. Would you comply with Mrs. S.'s request for the 'major breakthrough' penicillin?

3. Patients' needs are not synonymous with patients' demands. What factors govern the creation of patient expectations?
   a. If a doctor wishes to modify a patient's demands in the light of his professional assessment of the situation, what techniques are likely to achieve his objective?
   b. How would you cope with Mrs. S.'s demand?

J. D. E. Knox, Dundee

349 MR. C.C.E.   AGED 28   UNEMPLOYED

1. What determines someone's personality?
   a. Is personality purely inherited?
   b. Can low self esteem result from a physical disorder such as asthma? If so, how?
   c. Does personality often contribute to associations between unlikely diseases (such as asthma with urethritis)?
   d. What suggestions could be used to boost this patient's ego?

2. What constitutes patient compliance?
   a. Do GP's tend to think of compliance simply in terms of drug therapy?

b. What factors would have made this patient accept the use of fenoterol but not accept the use of beclomethasone and sodium cromoglycate?

c. Having been advised by a consultant to use both beclomethosone and sodium cromoglycate, how is the patient's compliance likely to be affected by the warning (printed in the GP's prescribing schedule) that the simultaneous use of beclomethasone and sodium cromoglycate is not recommended?

d. Have doctors any moral or ethical right to expect patients not to be promiscuous?

e. Have doctors any right to expect promiscuous patients to wear a condom?

f. Where alcohol abuse is controlled how much credit can the doctor claim in achieving compliance?

g. Where fenoterol abuse exists should compliance be achieved by refusing to prescribe the drug?

3. What prognostic factors are evident in this case?
   a. What are the prospects of changing a person's personality?
   b. Once an alcohol abuser, always an alcohol abuser?
   c. What is the relationship between compliance and prognosis in asthma?
   d. What is the likely outcome of a prescription supplied for amoxycillin 250 mg 8 hourly for a week?

D. Levet, Hobart

MR. H.D.   AGED 49   BUSINESS EXECUTIVE   **350**

1. What salient physical findings should be sought?
   a. Is the fact that the patient appears acutely ill of diagnostic significance?
   b. What diagnostic possibilities are entertained by finding dullness to percussion of the left base of the lung with bronchial breath sounds, both associated with increased vocal and tactile fremitus and rales in the left base?
   c. What positive diagnostic and prognostic considerations are suggested by the finding of generalized wheezing throughout both lungs with a prolonged expiratory phase?

2. What laboratory aids might be expected to offer positive diagnostic information?
   a. What is the significance of the blood culture revealing a Gram negative organism grown two days after plating?
   b. What is the significance of serum obtained on admission showing group B *Haemophilus influenzae* antigen on counter immunoelectrophoresis (CIE)? Is this helpful?

    c.   What are the differential diagnostic possibilities when the chest X-ray report reveals infiltration of the left lower lobe with some fluid in the left pleural cavity?

    d.   Does a Gram stain of the sputum help in determining immediate appropriate therapy?

3.   What are the most likely aetiological causes for secondary or post-influenzal pneumonia, more likely with underlying pulmonary disease such as asthma?

    a.   What changes are likely because of damage to the bronchial epithelium and transient impairment of normal pulmonary clearing mechanisms, such as cilia and mucus flow following influenza?

    b.   What factors make *Mycoplasma* infection unlikely as an aetiological agent in this patient?

    c.   What historical factors and diagnostic procedures would be helpful in ruling out pulmonary embolism in this case?

    d.   What further considerations are important, knowing that this patient has been on prednisone for five years as part of the therapy for asthma?

L. H. Amundson, Sioux Falls, SD, USA

351   MR. L.S.   AGED 62

1.   Does this patient suffer from bronchitis or asthma?

    a.   What investigations are available to help determine this?

    b.   Is a therapeutic trial of steroids justifiable even though reversible airways obstruction cannot be demonstrated?

2.   Discuss the management of late onset (intrinsic) asthma.

    a.   Could his occupation be relevant?

    b.   What drugs are available to combat bronchospasm: are these best delivered orally or by aerosol?

    c.   Discuss inhalation techniques and the various types of inhaler.

A. G. Strube, Crawley, UK

352   MRS. T.   AGED 23   BANK CLERK

1.   Why was the patient's illness initially refractory to treatment?

    a.   What is the medical management of bronchitis with bronchospasm?

    b.   Could allergy play a role in the response to treatment?

    c.   Could psychogenic factors play a role in the response to treatment?

d. What role does the severity of symptoms play in the response to treatment?
e. Is a change of antibiotic justified if there is an initial failure of response to treatment?

2. How would you manage this patient further?
    a. What role could the patient's smoking habits play in perpetuating her respiratory problems?
    b. How can the GP help the patient to reduce her cigarette smoking while also giving attention to her emotional state?
    c. To what extent, if any, should the GP give advice?
    d. What attitude should the GP adopt if the patient continues smoking?
    e. What is meant by non-judgmental acceptance?
    f. Of what value is the peak flow meter in assessing the patient's respiratory status?

S. Levenstein, Cape Town

MR. L.B.   AGED 52   353

1. How could the diagnosis have been made earlier?
    a. Would earlier intervention have influenced the final outcome?
    b. Could he have been treated at home?
    c. Does the involvement of three different doctors make management less effective?
    d. How can this be avoided?

2. What is meant by the term 'congestion'?
    a. Describe the signs in the lungs and heart which may occur in left ventricular failure.
    b. How may this be distinguished from asthmatic bronchitis?

A. G. Strube, Crawley, UK

MR. G.   AGED 32   FARMER   354

1. What further historical information is necessary to confirm the diagnosis?
    a. What details of style of farming are important in this man's history?
    b. What season of the year was this man likely to present in?
    c. What characteristic of the climate is this problem related to?

2. What further investigations would be helpful at this point in time? Even though a chest X-ray was done one month previously would a repeat chest X-ray be of benefit?

a. Would a complete blood count and differential be helpful in confirming the diagnosis?
b. Are there very specific blood tests that might be helpful in confirming this diagnosis in this situation?
c. What X-ray findings are most likely with the history?

3. Why have previous efforts to treat this man failed?
   a. Why do antibiotics not help in this situation?
   b. What is the treatment of choice in this situation?
   c. How rapidly would you expect a response to the treatment of choice?

W. W. Rosser, Ottawa

355 MR. PETER Z.   AGED 57   STOREMAN

1. What investigations would assist in diagnosis?
   a. Are you worried by the sudden onset of pneumonia, with no previous respiratory history?
   b. Is iron deficiency anaemia a contributory cause to pneumonia?
   c. Is further investigation of the respiratory tract necessary?
   d. Are further investigations of the anaemia necessary?

2. If all your investigations regarding the cause of the anaemia were negative, how would you manage the patient in the future?
   a. If expense were a problem in repeated investigation what would your priority be over the next 6 months?

R. M. Meyer, Johannesburg

356 MRS. BETINA A. & MR. HARRY A.   AGES: BETINA 42, HARRY 44
BETINA: HOUSEWIFE   HARRY: PANEL BEATER

1. What are some common causes of accelerated biological ageing?
   a. Is the comparison of chronological age and biological age a significant diagnostic process?
   b. How often do visual 'clues' play a role in clinical decision making?
   c. Are medical graduates trained to think of industrial toxins as a cause of ill-health?
   d. What industrial toxins can cause or aggravate obstructive lung disease?

2. What diagnoses are you considering at this stage?
   a. What cues triggered off the thoughts leading to your diagnostic postulates?

   b.   What conditions can you think of that can be diagnosed by simple observation?

   c.   How often do you need special investigations to confirm diagnoses made by observation?

3. Given that you have limited time available, how will you manage the consultation from this point onwards?

   a.   How do you manage a patient consultation where there is:
- a mixture of organic and psychological problems?
- more than one problem?

   b.   What is the significance of a spouse attending during a consultation with the other member of a marriage?

   c.   In your experience, how often would illness in a spouse produce this kind of domestic relationship?

   d.   What kind of illness in a spouse is commonly associated with this kind of husband–wife interaction?

M. W. Heffernan, Melbourne

MR. R.S.   AGED 38   TRUCK DRIVER   357

1. What does the family physician suspect as the aetiology at the first visit?

   a.   What clinical signs and symptoms support this?

   b.   Do you think he suspects a bacterial or viral aetiology?

   c.   If viral, do you think he would/should prescribe antibiotics?

   d.   How often do physicians prescribe antibiotics for chest infections which are suspected to be viral in origin?

   e.   Why do they do this; do you agree?

   f.   From what disease entity was this man suffering?

2. How commonly do patients suffer from occupational related diseases?

   a.   Are they usually, sometimes, or seldom recognized by family physicians?

   b.   Are physicians usually trained to recognize occupationally related diseases?

   c.   What resources are available to physicians with questions related to occupational health?

   d.   Do you believe pre-employment physicals are useful?

   e.   What is the role of an occupational hygienist?

3. What are the issues – ethical, moral and legal, relating to this man's concerns about reporting his disease?

   a.   Is it the doctor's moral responsibility to protect this man's job, or the other employees who may be similarly exposed?

b. Does the physician have a legal responsibility to override his patient's concerns and report this hazard?

c. What are the ethical implications to the physician in view of the source of his information, his patient being reluctant to have it revealed?

d. How should employees be protected from health risks in the workplace?

C. A. Moore, Hamilton, Canada

358 MR. B.P. AGED 18 FARM LABOURER

1. What additional information is required to reach a diagnosis?
   a. Would the taking of a complete family history be justified at this first urgent consultation?
   b. Should a traumatic cause be seriously considered?
   c. Is it important to know his state of health immediately prior to the football match?

2. What possible causes should be considered?
   a. What are the probabilities of this condition being skeletal in origin?
   b. Does the age of the patient exclude serious myocardial vascular disease?
   c. To establish early diagnosis in this case, which would be more important, the history, the examination, or any immediate investigations?

3. How should this patient be managed?
   a. Would an immediate ECG be likely to elucidate the problem?
   b. Should the patient be kept in the small hospital for observation or should he be transported to a larger base hospital?
   c. If there are ECG changes apparent suggesting myocardial vascular disease, what further investigations should be advised?
   d. How would you describe the prognosis to the patient?
   e. What preventive advice should be given?

T. D. Manthorpe, Port Lincoln, Australia

359 JOE SMITH AGED 33 ELECTRICIAN

1. What are the possible causes of his chest pain?
   a. Could this be cardiac ischaemia?
   b. What features suggest pulmonary chest pain?
   c. What other possible causes of this pain are there?

2. What investigations are indicated?

a. What information would an ECG give you?
b. How would X-rays help you?
c. Would any blood tests contribute anything?
d. Which tests are 'cost effective' on a Sunday afternoon?

3. What is this patient's main problem?
   a. What is a workaholic?
   b. Is this his only problem?
   c. How are others affected?

4. How would you manage this problem?
   a. How would specialist referral help?
   b. How might changes in life style be achieved?
   c. In what way should his wife and family be involved?
   d. What opportunities are there for health promotion?

R. P. Strasser, Melbourne

MR. M.T.   AGED 31   CLERK   360

1. What diagnostic possibilities would you consider whilst driving to the patient's home?
   a. Which of these conditions is life-threatening?
   b. What action would you take?
   c. What is the place of a mobile resuscitation unit (coronary ambulance) in the management of acute chest pain outside of the hospital?

2. Why might he be hyperventilating?
   a. What are the effects of hyperventilation?
   b. Why should he have incipient tetany?
   c. How would you demonstrate this?
   d. How would you manage the situation?

3. What factors tend to make relatives particularly anxious about a patient's condition?
   a. How would you explore the underlying problems in this case?
   b. How can you be sure that you are 'reassuring' the patient and family rather than yourself?

E. C. Gambrill, Crawley, UK

JOHN ROBERTS   AGED 48   COMPANY MANAGER   361

1. What is the problem in this case?
   a. Despite the normal ECG, could this be cardiac ischaemia?
   b. Describe the features of an acute anxiety attack?
   c. What is 'cardiac neurosis'?

2. Are any further investigations indicated?
   a. How would any further tests help you?
   b. Would further investigations help the patient?
   c. Would specialist referral help at this stage?

3. How would you manage this problem?
   a. What medications are indicated?
   b. Will the problem be resolved with just one consultation?
   c. Who else might you involve in managing this case?
   d. What opportunity does this event present for health promotion and preventive care?

R. P. Strasser, Melbourne

362 MRS. S.S.   AGED 45   CLERICAL WORKER

1. What is your differential diagnosis for the emergency consultation?
   a. What are the advantages and disadvantages of hospital admission for myocardial infarction in patients without shock or cardiac arrhythmia?
   b. What do you know about costochrondrosis and its management?
   c. What are the possible clinical findings when a patient complains of palpitations?

2. What is your problem list for Mrs. S.S.?
   a. What do you know about associations between hysterectomy and emotional state?
   b. What are your criteria for the diagnosis of spastic colon?
   c. What do you understand by the term 'random association' and give clinical examples of it?

3. What are your criteria for giving anti-depressant medication?
   a. What are the common stages of bereavement experience and their duration?
   b. Is anti-depressant medication ever justified for recently bereaved people?
   c. What are the side-effects of the commonly used anti-depressants? Do these side-effects alter with dosage or duration of treatment?

P. Freeling, London

363 MR. M.F.   AGED 59   RETIRED CLERK

1. What are the aetiological factors in this man's myocardial infarction?
   a. What are the risk factors for myocardial infarction?

    b.   What is the role of the beta-blocker in the prevention/diminution of the size of a myocardial infarct?

2. What is your management of this situation?
    a.   How would you provide pain relief to this man?
    b.   Does an anti-arrhythmic have a place in this situation?
    c.   How do you organize the transfer of this man to hospital (if that is your plan of management)?
    d.   What would you include in your explanation to this man's wife?

D. S. Pedler, Adelaide

HAROLD O'HALLORAN   AGED 85   PENSIONER   **364**

1. How do you explain the episode of agitation and confusion three years ago?
    a.   Could pneumonia alone cause such an episode?
    b.   How does senile dementia affect people?
    c.   Might hospital admission itself have contributed?
    d.   What is 'acute brain syndrome'?

2. Is hospital admission indicated this time?
    a.   Would you (cardiac) monitor this patient?
    b.   What are the advantages of hospital treatment?
    c.   What disadvantage might there be with hospital treatment?

3. Could you manage this patient at home?
    a.   Is family support sufficient to manage his medications and recognize any sudden change in his condition?
    b.   How could the district nurse help?
    c.   With frequent home visits by you, how would his medical care differ at home from that in hospital?
    d.   Who else in the community might you involve?

R. P. Strasser, Melbourne

MR. M.S.   AGED 42   **365**

1. What are the diagnostic possibilities you would consider?
    a.   How can you exclude the more serious causes?

2. What other information would you wish to obtain to arrive at a more precise diagnosis?
    a.   What other factors in the history would you enquire about?
    b.   What investigations, if any, would you perform?
    c.   What physical signs would you look for?

3. How do you exclude a diagnosis of ischaemic disease in a young man?
   a. What features in the history enable you to arrive at a diagnosis?
   b. What physical signs would support such a diagnosis?
   c. What investigations can you perform? What are the indications and risks?
   d. What else can help you to confirm a diagnosis of angina? Would a trial of a drug for angina help?

4. In a patient with proven ischaemic heart disease, when do you refer him to a consultant?
   a. What are the indications for surgery in ischaemic heart disease?

H. C. Watts, Perth, Australia

366 MR. K.W. AGED 38 BUSINESSMAN

1. What is the significance of his chest pain?
   a. Is there anything else you should do to elicit the cause?
   b. If it is not cardiac in origin what might it be?
   c. How can the physician take advantage of his present symptoms to his benefit?

2. What are the most important risk factors in cardiovascular disease?
   a. Should you treat his blood pressure?
   b. Does lowering the BP improve the prognosis in cardiovascular disease?
   c. What should you do about his hypercholesterolaemia?
   d. What should you do about his smoking and alcohol intake?

3. What should you do about his other risk factors?
   a. What are the effects of stress on cardiovascular disease?
   b. What are the signs of stress?
   c. Would a change of lifestyle alter this man's chances of developing cardiovascular disease?

W. F. Glastonbury, Adelaide

367 MR. L.P. AGED 54 CLERGYMAN

1. How do you decide if chest pain is serious?
   a. Is the history or physical examination more important?
   b. Does a normal physical examination exclude serious disease?
   c. Is it safe to make a diagnosis of benign chest wall pain by exclusion only?

2. What diagnostic tests help?
   a. Is the ECG always abnormal?
   b. Does a chest X-ray often give helpful information?
   c. What is the timing of cardiac enzyme changes?
   d. What about a therapeutic trial of nitroglycerine?
   e. What other tests do you order if the cardiac investigation is negative?
   f. When would you perform an exercise ECG?

3. What counselling do you give to the patient with coronary artery disease and to his family?
   a. What is the appropriate timing of such advice?
   b. Do you always say the same thing to the patient and to the family?
   c. How important is diet?
   d. How do you prescribe an exercise program?
   e. How soon can a 'heart' patient resume sexual activity?
   f. What psychological problems may you encounter after the patient returns home?
   g. How do you decide when the patient can resume work?

R. L. Perkin, Toronto

MRS. C.D.   AGED 55   HOUSEWIFE   **368**

1. What is the cause of the pain?
   a. What other physical sign might develop in the next 48 hours to help clarify the diagnosis?
   b. Does the diagnosis depend on this sign?
   c. If this sign develops, will it be possible to make an exact diagnosis?

2. What place have corticosteroids in the treatment of this patient?
   a. Will corticosteroids ease the pain?
   b. Will corticosteroids interfere with the patient's immune response in relation to the malignancy or the cause of the pain?
   c. How often should this patient be reviewed?

3. How much of this patient's illness has been due to cigarette smoking?
   a. In what way would the course of her illnesses be altered by the immediate cessation of smoking?
   b. Would reduction but not cessation of smoking be beneficial?
   c. How can a general practitioner assist a person who wants to stop smoking?

B. H. Connor, Armidale, Australia

369   MR. A.W.   AGED 31   CLERK

1. How would you manage his clinical problem?
   a. How would you treat him medically?
   b. What are the risks in coronary arteriography?
   c. What are the indications for a coronary bypass operation?

2. How do you prevent the patient from becoming a cardiac invalid?
   a. How would you advise him regarding exercise and sexual relations?
   b. What is his prognosis?

3. How would his problem affect his family and his community?
   a. What is your approach in informing his wife of his condition?
   b. What are the community resources available for such a cardiac patient in your community?

F. E. H. Tan, Kuala Lumpur

370   WALTER M.   AGED 45   STOREMAN

1. What diagnostic suspicions should these findings arouse in the doctor's mind?
   a. What special information could the radiologist be expected to provide in his report on the fractured ribs?
   b. What particular physical findings should be sought by the doctor in the light of the patient's presentation?
   c. What tests should the doctor now select in order to make the diagnosis?

2. What is the most likely cause of Walter M.'s rib fracture?
   a. Apart from X-raying the ribs what other X-ray could be ordered that would clinch the diagnosis?
   b. What would be the significance of a raised blood urea?
   c. What would be the value of a protein electrophoretogram (EPG)?
   d. Would an EPG be of diagnostic value on any other body fluids?
   e. What, if any, diagnostic findings would the pathologist expect from bone marrow biopsy?

3. What matters should the family doctor discuss with the patient and his family?
   a. Who should be present at these discussions?
   b. How should the doctor respond if asked the question – 'Is it cancer?'
   c. How should the doctor respond if asked the question – 'Am I going to die?'

W. L. Ogborne, Sydney

MR. T.S.   AGED 45   BUSINESS EXECUTIVE   **371**

1. What is your differential diagnosis?
   a. What are the possible presenting features of carcinoma of the bronchus?
   b. What are your criteria for the diagnosis of chronic bronchitis?
   c. What features of a patient's history might lead you to suspect alcohol abuse?
   d. What disorders might present with bruising?

2. Which one diagnosis would most logically explain all the features of this patient's history and examination?
   a. What blood tests would help to substantiate a diagnosis of chronic alcohol abuse?
   b. Describe the progression of the alcoholic from social drinking to chronic alcohol dependence.
   c. What methods and agencies are available to help the chronic alcoholic?
   d. What are the features of the alcohol withdrawal syndrome?

3. To what aspects of the history and examination would you pay particular attention in carrying out a routine check-up on a 45 year old man?
   a. With what conditions is cigarette smoking associated?
   b. How would you advise a patient who wished to give up smoking?
   c. Devise an exercise plan for a middle-aged man who has led a sedentary life for the past ten years.
   d. What measures would you take if you found a 45 year old man to have a BP of 160/105?

T. A. I. Bouchier Hayes, Camberley, UK

MISS P.C.   AGED 25   OFFICE CLEANER   **372**

1. What are the likely diagnoses here?
   a. Is the infection likely to be viral or bacterial?

2. What investigations would you undertake?
   a. What would you expect on chest X-ray?
   b. What would you expect on blood film examination?

3. Does a negative chest X-ray alter your diagnosis?

4. What is the significance of her statement that her father died from lung cancer?

    a.   How would you help her anxiety in relation to her present illness?

    b.   How would you help her anxiety in relation to her father's death from lung cancer?

D. U. Shepherd, Melbourne

373   MRS. J.P.   AGED 51   HOUSEWIFE

1. What is the pathogen?
   a. How many types of *Pneumococcus* are identified?
   b. How are they distinguished from each other?
   c. What is the quickest method of making the diagnosis?
   d. What will the chest X-ray show at the beginning, and later on?
   e. What pre-existing conditions are often present in patients with pneumococcal infection?

2. How would you treat the patient?
   a. What dose of penicillin is appropriate?
   b. What alternative drugs can you use if the patient is allergic to penicillin?
   c. How long would you treat the patient?
   d. Is type specific pneumococcal antiserum ever used? If so, in what circumstances?

3. What preventive measures would you advise for the future?
   a. Is it important for the patient to stop smoking?
   b. Does one bout of pneumococcal pneumonia confer lifelong immunity?
   c. Would you give the patient pneumococcal vaccine (Pneumovax)?
   d. How often does the patient need booster doses of Pneumovax?

R. L. Perkin, Toronto

374   MR. B.F.   AGED 44   PLANT WORKER

1. What are the essential problems and their differential diagnosis?
   a. Chest pain?
   b. Dyspnoea?
   c. Hypertension?
   d. Past history of thrombophlebitis?

2. What are the possible risk factors to be considered in this case?
   a. Would a history of moderate smoking be significant?
   b. What specific family history should be obtained?

   c.   Would a history of previous response to anti-hypertensive medication have any bearing on the differential diagnosis of hypertension?

   d.   Would it be important to obtain a history of any trauma, immobilization or surgery, as well as the work habits of this plant worker?

   e.   What drug related complications might be expected during the therapy of this patient?

       a.   What are the main complications of heparin and coumarin?

       b.   What side effects might be observed from the use of diuretics and digitalis?

       c.   What complications might be expected from the diagnostic use of lymphangiography, venography, and Doppler ultrasound?

   f.   What chronic changes can occur in the leg from repeated thrombophlebitis?

   g.   How might his diagnosis and therapy influence his job description upon return to work?

L. H. Amundson, Sioux Falls, SD, USA

MR. K.   AGED 45   BANK CLERK   **375**

1. What was the first GP's diagnosis?

   a.   How can one distinguish between chest pain of cardiac and non-cardiac origin?

   b.   What are the commoner non-cardiac causes of chest pain in general practice?

   c.   To what extent may the patient's previous cardiovascular status have influenced the GP's initial assessment?

2. Why was the patient so anxious at the consultation with the 'locum' GP?

   a.   Was the effect of the first GP's 'reassurance' cancelled out by the 'double-message' of being told to go to bed for 3 days?

   b.   How effective is reassurance in allaying patients' anxieties?

   c.   To what extent may the patient's anxiety have been due to his regular GP having gone on leave at that time?

   d.   To what extent may the patient's anxiety have been unrelated to his present symptoms?

3. Why was the patient relieved after the consultation with the 'locum' GP?

   a.   To what extent is the use of an ECG to reassure a patient justified?

   b.   Was the patient reassured by being told he could return to work the next day?

   c. Was the GP justified in telling the patient he could return to work the next day?
   d. Is the patient likely to remain 'reassured' for long?
   e. Is the patient likely to develop chest pain again?
   f. If the patient does develop chest pain and/or anxiety symptoms again, how should the GP manage the situation?

S. Levenstein, Cape Town

376   MR. C.H.   AGED 57   LABOURER

1. What syndrome does Mr. H.'s story illustrate?
   a. What are the characteristics of angina?
   b. What investigations would you undertake if you suspected ischaemic heart disease? How would you advise a patient who displays cardiac neurosis?
   d. Design a protocol for the differential diagnosis of chest pain.

2. What are the reasons for frequent office attendance by a patient with no evidence of physical disease?
   a. What do you understand by the concept of 'the doctor as treatment'?
   b. What strategies might you use to end a consultation when useful communication has finished?
   c. What do you feel about the doctor's role as counsellor?
   d. Of what significance is physical contact between doctor and patient?

3. What resources are available for the health education of patients?
   a. How can the various members of the primary care team contribute towards health education in the practice?
   b. What problems may be caused by media coverage of medical topics?
   c. What subjects would you cover if asked to speak to a lay audience on the topic of ischaemic heart disease?

T. A. I. Bouchier Hayes, Camberley, UK

377   MRS. S.H.   AGED 40   HOUSEWIFE/SOCIAL WORKER

1. What investigations might be indicated at this most recent visit?
   a. Is it possible that repeated investigations might be 'reinforcing the illness' in the mind of the patient?
   b. What new historical or objective data might cause you to re-investigate the symptoms?

2. What referral(s) might be indicated at this most recent visit?
   a. Is it possible that repeated referrals might be 'reinforcing the illness' in the mind of the patient?
   b. What new historical or objective data might cause you to again refer this patient to a consultant physician?
   c. Is it likely that referral to a psychiatrist would be useful?

3. What is the most likely cause of this patient's symptoms?
   a. What are some of the clinical features of angina pectoris?
   b. What are some of the clinical features of hyperventilation related to anxiety?
   c. What are some of the clinical features of cardiac neurosis?

G. G. Beazley, Winnipeg

MR. J.P.   AGED 53   EXECUTIVE   378

1. What would be your strategies for dealing with such an obviously complex problem in a busy consulting session?
   a. Given plenty of time how would you proceed from the initial history above?

2. How can you distinguish between the various causes of retrosternal and epigastric pain?
   a. What characteristics of history do you recognize?
   b. What physical signs may help in your differential diagnosis?
   c. What tests may help?

3. What would you do if you're not sure of the diagnosis even if you have sought another opinion?

F. Mansfield, Perth, Australia

LES B.   AGED 32   SALESMAN   379

1. What is the single most likely process by which Les B.'s symptoms will be diagnosed?
   a. What fundamentals of history taking must be observed if the diagnostic clues are to be recognized?
   b. What anatomical considerations should govern the clinician's approach to chest pain around the left breast?
   c. What simple diagnostic manoeuvres can be employed in the consulting room in order to identify the cause of Les B.'s chest pain?

2. Why have so many doctors failed to diagnose the cause of Les B.'s chest pain?
   a. What factors inherent in the medical consultation hinder the diagnostic process?
   b. How does the doctor's perception of his professional role influence the diagnostic process?

3. During physical examination the spinous processes of T3 and T4 are very tender when firm pressure is applied with the thumb. What relationship, if any, does this finding have to Les B.'s chest pain?
   a. Is the tenderness to pressure on the spinous processes T3 and T4 compatible with any elements of Les B.'s history?
   b. What simple procedure can be performed in the consulting room to relieve Les B. of his chest pain?
   c. How is this procedure performed?
   d. What advice should be given to Les B. regarding recurrence of his chest pain?
   e. What factors will determine whether or not such recurrences will occur?

W. L. Ogborne, Sydney

380   DESMOND K.   AGED 58   FACTORY MANAGER

1. What are the characteristics of the pain of angina pectoris?
   a. What instructions and explanation should be given at the time the glyceryl trinitrate was prescribed?
   b. What other drug therapy might have been given in this case?
   c. What other causes of retrosternal pain must be considered in the differential diagnosis?
   d. What general advice should this patient have been given at the initial consultation?

2. What action should the general practitioner take in relation to the patient's complaints at the most recent consultation?
   a. What are the possible advantages and disadvantages of a conservative approach?
   b. How important is the general practitioner in improving the statistics dealing with morbidity and mortality from common diseases?
   c. What further treatments may be available to this patient, what success has been achieved, and what are the social and economic implications of making these treatments increasingly available?

J. G. P. Ryan, Brisbane

MR. M.N.   AGED 41   FORK HOIST DRIVER   # 381

1. How should Dr. Y. advise the patient?
   a. What are his responsibilities for making sure that the patient is handed back to his family doctor?
   b. How does he make it clear that it is Dr. Y.'s duty to inform the locum tenens of his interest in the patient's ability to work and any proposed treatment which may affect his working performance?

2. How should Dr. Y. advise the employer?
   a. What is the nature of the relationship between an industrial medical officer and the company for whom he works?
   b. Is there any change in the nature of the doctor's duty towards the patient?
   c. If this patient refuses to allow the doctor to discuss his medical condition with officials of the firm, what does the doctor do next?

3. What should Dr. Y. do with regard to the patient's own doctor's locum?
   a. What do you know about established rules for ethical practice of medicine by industrial medical officers?

P. L. Gibson, Auckland

THOMAS D.   AGED 52   COMPANY EXECUTIVE   # 382

1. How would you manage the continuing care of his angina and transient ischaemic attacks?
   a. What drugs are useful in these conditions?
   b. What should the patient be told about his prognosis?

2. How would you react to the decision preventing him from driving a car?
   a. What kind of feelings might it arouse in the patient?
   b. What role should the doctor adopt?

3. What responsibility does the general practitioner have in the prevention of arterial disease?
   a. What are the main predisposing factors for ischaemic heart disease and stroke?
   b. Can the doctor influence any of these factors?
   c. Should he attempt to do so?
   d. What would be the implications in terms of time and resources?

J. C. Hasler, Oxford

383

MR. W.R.   AGED 65

1. Are coronary heart disease and peripheral vascular disease related?
    a. What are the predisposing factors?
    b. What actual pathological features are involved?
    c. Why does propranolol help angina but aggravate peripheral disease?
    d. Why does glyceryl trinitrate help angina but not peripheral disease?

2. What is the basis for this patient's hypertension?
    a. If a patient has rigid blood vessels and an ischaemic myocardium, what treatment is rational for the blood pressure?
    b. What are the fundamental effects of beta-blocking drugs in hypertension?
    c. What is the rationale for trying a cardio-selective beta-blocking agent in this case?
    d. How does prazosin work in hypertension? Is it more suitable than beta-blockers?

3. Is it rational to treat this patient's blood pressure?
    a. What is the risk of stroke if blood pressure is treated or untreated?
    b. How does one explain to the patient that one is treating the blood pressure and not the ischaemic heart disease. Does this distinction matter?

A. L. A. Reid, Newcastle, Australia